REVENUE CYCLE MANAGEMENT

-

One Book To Make You Genius

by

VIRUTI SHIVAN

"Embark on a Thriving Career in Revenue Cycle Management:

Unleash Your Potential, Drive Financial Success"

Starting a career in revenue cycle management is like embarking on an exciting journey, where every challenge you encounter becomes an opportunity for growth, and every success brings you closer to financial success. As you navigate the ins and outs of revenue cycle management, remember that your knowledge and expertise will be your guide. By dedicating yourself to learning and understanding the revenue cycle, you have the power to improve financial operations and make a meaningful impact in healthcare. Embrace this journey, take charge of your career, and witness the incredible potential that revenue cycle management holds for you.

Preface

Revenue cycle management (RCM) plays a vital role in the financial health and sustainability of healthcare organizations. It encompasses a complex array of processes, from patient registration to claim adjudication and payment collection. The effective management of these processes ensures accurate and timely reimbursement for services rendered, reduces claim denials, and enhances overall revenue optimization.

This comprehensive guide on revenue cycle management aims to provide students, practitioners, and healthcare professionals with a thorough understanding of the principles, best practices, and strategies involved in optimizing the revenue cycle. Whether you are a novice seeking to grasp the fundamentals or an experienced professional aiming to enhance your expertise, this guide covers a wide range of topics, offering a step-by-step journey from the basics to mastery-level understanding.

The guide begins by introducing the revenue cycle and its significance in the healthcare industry. It then delves into various aspects of revenue cycle management, such as patient pre-registration, appointment scheduling, medical coding and documentation, claims submission, denial management, patient billing, compliance, technology integration, performance measurement, and much more.

To ensure practical applicability, each chapter incorporates real-life case studies, examples, exercises, and scenarios that allow readers to connect theoretical concepts to real-world situations. Additionally, the appendix provides a wealth of useful resources, including glossaries, recommended books, online courses, professional associations, industry publications, compliance guidelines, and certification programs, to further enrich the learning experience.

We understand that revenue cycle management is an ever-evolving field, influenced by changes in technology, regulations, and industry trends. Therefore, this guide encourages continuous learning and adaptation to stay abreast of the latest developments in RCM.

We hope this comprehensive guide serves as a valuable resource, empowering you to navigate the intricacies of revenue cycle management with confidence and proficiency. Whether you are a student embarking on a career in healthcare administration or a seasoned professional seeking to optimize revenue operations, this guide equips you with the knowledge and tools necessary to succeed in today's dynamic healthcare landscape.

Remember, revenue cycle management is a collaborative effort that requires effective communication, interdisciplinary coordination, and a commitment to delivering quality care while ensuring financial stability. Together, let us embark on this journey of understanding and mastering revenue cycle management.

Best regards,

VIRUTI SHIVAN

Table of Contents

1. Introduction to Revenue Cycle Management

1.1 Definition and Overview of Revenue Cycle Management:

Revenue cycle management (RCM) refers to the strategic management and optimization of the financial processes involved in a healthcare organization's revenue cycle. It encompasses a wide range of administrative and clinical activities aimed at ensuring accurate and timely reimbursement for services rendered to patients.

The revenue cycle starts when a patient seeks medical services and continues through the entire billing and payment process until all outstanding balances are resolved. RCM involves coordinating various stages of the revenue cycle, including patient registration, coding and documentation, claims submission, payment posting, and patient billing and collections.

The primary objective of RCM is to maximize revenue collection while minimizing inefficiencies and reducing claim denials. By implementing effective RCM practices, healthcare organizations can streamline their revenue processes, improve cash flow, optimize reimbursements, and enhance financial stability.

Overview of Revenue Cycle Management:

1. Patient Registration: The revenue cycle begins with patient registration, where demographic and insurance information is collected. This step ensures accurate patient identification, verifies insurance coverage, and establishes a financial account.

2. Coding and Documentation: Healthcare providers document the services provided using standardized codes such as Current Procedural Terminology (CPT) and International Classification of Diseases (ICD). Accurate coding and documentation are essential for proper billing and claims submission.

3. Charge Capture: This step involves capturing charges associated with the services provided, including procedures, supplies, and medications. Accurate charge capture ensures that all billable services are appropriately recorded for reimbursement.

4. Claims Submission: Once services are documented and charges are captured, healthcare organizations submit claims to insurance companies or payers for reimbursement. Claims are submitted electronically using standardized formats such as HIPAA-compliant electronic data interchange (EDI) formats.

5. Claims Adjudication: After receiving claims, insurance companies or payers review them for accuracy and process them. This step involves verifying patient eligibility, reviewing the services provided, and determining the appropriate reimbursement based on the payer's fee schedule or contractual agreements.

6. Payment Posting: Once claims are adjudicated, insurance companies provide reimbursement to healthcare organizations. Payment posting involves recording the payment received, adjusting the patient's account, and reconciling any discrepancies.

7. Patient Billing and Collections: After insurance reimbursement, patients are billed for their portion of the healthcare services, including copayments, deductibles, and any outstanding balances. Effective patient billing and collections processes ensure timely payment from patients.

By effectively managing each stage of the revenue cycle, healthcare organizations can optimize revenue collection, reduce claim denials, enhance cash flow, and improve financial performance.

1.2 Importance and Benefits of Effective RCM:

Effective revenue cycle management (RCM) is crucial for the financial health and success of healthcare organizations. Here are some key reasons why RCM is of paramount importance:

a. Financial Stability: A well-managed revenue cycle ensures the financial stability of healthcare organizations. By optimizing revenue collection, organizations can cover their expenses, invest in technology and infrastructure, and support quality patient care.

b. Timely Reimbursement: Efficient RCM processes expedite the reimbursement cycle, ensuring that healthcare providers receive timely payment for their services. This improves cash flow and reduces financial strain, allowing organizations to meet their financial obligations and fund operational needs.

c. Reduced Claim Denials: Effective RCM practices help minimize claim denials, which can significantly impact revenue. By implementing robust processes, including accurate coding and documentation, eligibility verification, and claims scrubbing, healthcare organizations can proactively identify and address potential issues that could lead to claim denials. This reduces the need for rework, speeds up reimbursement, and maximizes revenue.

d. Enhanced Revenue Optimization: RCM enables organizations to identify areas of revenue leakage and optimize revenue collection. By closely monitoring and analyzing key performance indicators (KPIs) such as clean claim rates, days in accounts receivable, and collection rates, organizations can pinpoint bottlenecks, implement process improvements, and negotiate favorable contracts with payers. These actions can lead to increased revenue capture and improved financial performance.

e. Improved Patient Satisfaction: Effective RCM processes contribute to a smoother billing and collections experience for patients. Clear and transparent communication of financial responsibilities, accurate billing statements, and efficient handling of inquiries and disputes enhance patient satisfaction. Positive patient experiences foster trust, loyalty, and positive word-of-mouth referrals, benefiting the organization's reputation and future revenue potential.

f. Compliance and Risk Mitigation: Adhering to regulatory requirements and industry standards in RCM helps healthcare organizations mitigate compliance risks and avoid penalties. Compliance with regulations such as the Health Insurance Portability and Accountability Act (HIPAA) safeguards patient data privacy and protects the organization's reputation.

g. Data-Driven Decision Making: RCM provides organizations with valuable financial data and analytics. By tracking and analyzing RCM metrics, organizations can gain insights into their financial performance, identify trends, and make informed decisions. Data-driven decision making allows organizations to implement targeted strategies for revenue optimization and process improvement.

Overall, effective RCM is essential for maintaining financial stability, ensuring timely reimbursement, reducing claim denials, enhancing patient satisfaction, mitigating compliance risks, and enabling data-driven decision making. By investing in RCM processes, technology, and training, healthcare organizations can optimize their revenue cycles and achieve long-term financial success.

1.3 Key Players in the Revenue Cycle:

The revenue cycle involves collaboration among various stakeholders who play critical roles in ensuring its smooth operation and financial success. Here are the key players involved in revenue cycle management (RCM):

1. Healthcare Providers: Healthcare providers, including physicians, nurses, therapists, and other clinical staff, are at the forefront of delivering patient care. They play a crucial role in documenting patient encounters, providing accurate diagnoses, and ensuring proper coding and documentation for billing purposes.

2. Administrative Staff: Administrative staff, such as front desk personnel, registration specialists, and billing and coding staff, are responsible for tasks related to patient registration, insurance verification, charge capture, claims submission, and patient billing. They ensure accurate and complete information is collected and processed throughout the revenue cycle.

3. Revenue Cycle Management Team: Organizations often have dedicated teams responsible for revenue cycle management. These teams typically include revenue cycle managers, analysts, coders, and billing specialists who oversee the end-to-end revenue cycle processes, analyze performance metrics, identify areas for improvement, and implement strategies to optimize revenue collection and minimize denials.

4. Payers: Payers, including private insurance companies, government payers (such as Medicare and Medicaid), and self-funded employers, play a significant role in the revenue cycle. They provide insurance coverage, determine reimbursement rates, process and adjudicate claims, and make payments to healthcare providers. Collaborating effectively with payers is crucial for accurate claims submission and timely reimbursement.

5. Patients: Patients are an essential component of the revenue cycle. They provide personal and insurance information during the registration process, seek medical services, and are responsible for their financial obligations. Effective communication with patients regarding insurance coverage, copayments, deductibles, and billing inquiries is crucial for successful revenue cycle management.

6. Technology and Software Providers: Technology plays a crucial role in streamlining revenue cycle processes. Electronic Health Record (EHR) systems, practice management software, billing and coding software, and revenue cycle management platforms automate and optimize various tasks, such as appointment scheduling, claims submission, coding, and billing. Technology vendors and software providers support organizations in implementing and maintaining these systems.

7. Regulatory and Compliance Bodies: Regulatory agencies and compliance bodies, such as the Centers for Medicare and Medicaid Services (CMS), the Office for Civil Rights (OCR), and state healthcare departments, establish guidelines and regulations that govern revenue cycle practices. Compliance with these regulations, including HIPAA, ensures patient data privacy, ethical billing practices, and accurate reporting.

8. Professional Associations and Industry Organizations: Professional associations and industry organizations, such as the Healthcare Financial Management Association (HFMA), the American Association of Professional Coders (AAPC), and regional or state-level healthcare organizations, offer resources, education, certifications, and networking opportunities to support revenue cycle professionals and promote industry best practices.

Collaboration and effective communication among these key players are essential for seamless revenue cycle management. Each stakeholder contributes to specific stages of the revenue cycle, and their coordination ensures accurate billing, timely reimbursement, and overall financial success for healthcare organizations.

Exercise 1: Introduction to Revenue Cycle Management

1. Definition and Overview of Revenue Cycle Management

Question 1: Define revenue cycle management (RCM) in the healthcare industry.

Answer: Revenue cycle management (RCM) refers to the strategic process of managing all administrative and clinical functions related to capturing, managing, and collecting revenue for healthcare services. It encompasses the entire revenue cycle, starting from patient registration to final payment, and involves various activities such as patient access, coding, billing, claims management, and reimbursement.

Question 2: List the key components of the revenue cycle.

Answer: The key components of the revenue cycle include:

- Patient registration and demographic data collection

- Insurance verification and eligibility checking

- Patient financial responsibility and estimation

- Scheduling and patient access management

- Medical coding and documentation

- Charge capture and reimbursement

- Claims submission and adjudication

- Denial management and appeals

- Insurance follow-up and accounts receivable management

- Patient billing and collections

2. Importance and Benefits of Effective RCM

Question 1: Explain why effective revenue cycle management is crucial for healthcare organizations.

Answer: Effective revenue cycle management is crucial for healthcare organizations due to the following reasons:

- Financial Stability: It ensures timely and accurate reimbursement for services rendered, helping to maintain financial stability and meet operational expenses.

- Optimized Revenue: Effective RCM processes help maximize revenue capture and minimize revenue leakage, resulting in increased financial performance.

- Compliance: RCM ensures compliance with regulatory requirements and coding guidelines, reducing the risk of audits, penalties, and legal issues.

- Patient Satisfaction: Streamlined RCM processes lead to accurate billing and transparent financial communication, improving patient satisfaction and loyalty.

- Operational Efficiency: Efficient RCM processes minimize claim denials, reduce billing errors, and enhance overall operational efficiency.

- Decision-Making: RCM provides valuable financial data and analytics, enabling informed decision-making and strategic planning for the organization.

3. Key Players in the Revenue Cycle

Question 1: Identify the key players involved in the revenue cycle management process.

Answer: The key players in the revenue cycle management process include:

- Patients: They are the recipients of healthcare services and have a role in providing accurate demographic and insurance information, as well as understanding their financial responsibilities.

- Front-end Staff: This includes registration personnel, schedulers, and patient access staff who collect patient information, verify insurance coverage, and estimate patient financial responsibility.

- Clinical Staff: Healthcare providers play a role in accurate and detailed documentation of medical services provided during patient encounters.

- Coding and Billing Staff: They are responsible for assigning appropriate codes to procedures and diagnoses, ensuring accurate and compliant billing, and submitting claims to payers.

- Payers: Insurance companies and government programs are involved in the reimbursement process by adjudicating claims and providing payment based on the terms of the insurance policy or program.

- Revenue Cycle Team: This team includes revenue cycle managers, analysts, and specialists who oversee and manage the entire revenue cycle process, ensuring efficiency, compliance, and financial performance.

These exercises provide an opportunity to reinforce the knowledge gained from the chapter on Introduction to Revenue Cycle Management. The questions assess understanding and reinforce key concepts related to the definition and overview of RCM, the importance and benefits of effective RCM, and the key players involved in the revenue cycle process.

2. Revenue Cycle Basics

2.1 Revenue Cycle Components and Workflow:

The revenue cycle in healthcare consists of various interconnected components and a sequential workflow that spans from the initial patient encounter to the final payment collection. Understanding the components and workflow of the revenue cycle is crucial for effective revenue cycle management. Let's explore each component and its role in the revenue cycle workflow:

1. Patient Scheduling:

The revenue cycle begins with patient scheduling, where appointments are booked for medical services. This stage involves coordinating patient preferences, provider availability, and necessary resources. Efficient scheduling practices help optimize resource utilization and ensure a smooth flow of patients through the revenue cycle.

2. Patient Registration:

Patient registration is the process of gathering necessary information from patients, including personal details, insurance information, and consent forms. Accurate and complete registration ensures proper patient identification, verifies insurance coverage, and establishes the financial account for billing and reimbursement purposes.

3. Eligibility Verification:

Eligibility verification is the process of confirming a patient's insurance coverage and benefits. It involves validating insurance details, checking co-pays, deductibles, and authorizations. Verifying eligibility upfront helps avoid claim denials and ensures accurate financial estimation and patient billing.

4. Point of Service Collections:

Point of Service (POS) collections involve collecting patient financial responsibilities, such as co-pays, deductibles, and co-insurance, at the time of service. Collecting payments upfront reduces bad debt and improves cash flow. Clear communication with patients regarding their financial obligations is essential during this stage.

5. Charge Capture:

Charge capture refers to the process of capturing and recording the charges associated with the services provided to the patient. It involves documenting procedures, supplies, medications, and other billable items accurately. Proper charge capture ensures that all billable services are accounted for in the subsequent billing and claims submission processes.

6. Coding and Documentation:

Coding and documentation are critical components of the revenue cycle. Medical coders review clinical documentation and assign appropriate codes using standardized code sets such as Current Procedural Terminology (CPT) and International Classification of Diseases (ICD). Accurate coding ensures proper billing, supports claims submission, and facilitates reimbursement.

7. Claims Submission:

Once the services are coded and documented, claims are submitted to insurance companies or payers for reimbursement. Claims submission involves compiling and transmitting all relevant information, including patient details, coded procedures, and supporting documentation, using standardized electronic formats such as HIPAA-compliant electronic data interchange (EDI).

8. Claims Adjudication:

Claims adjudication is the process where insurance companies or payers review and process the submitted claims. They assess the claims for accuracy, validity, and compliance with reimbursement policies. Adjudication involves eligibility verification, medical necessity review, fee schedule or contract analysis, and determination of reimbursement amounts.

9. Payment Posting:

After claims are adjudicated, insurance companies provide reimbursement to healthcare organizations. Payment posting involves recording the payment received, applying it to the patient's account, and reconciling any discrepancies. Accurate payment posting ensures proper account management and reconciliation of payments received.

10. Denial Management:

Denial management is the process of identifying and resolving claim denials. When a claim is denied, it is necessary to investigate the reason for denial, correct any errors or missing information, and resubmit the claim or file an appeal if necessary. Effective denial management minimizes revenue loss and ensures timely reimbursement.

11. Patient Billing and Collections:

Patient billing is the process of generating invoices or statements for the patient's portion of the healthcare services. This includes co-pays, deductibles, co-insurance, and any remaining balances after insurance reimbursement. Patient collections involve communicating the billing details to patients, managing payment plans, and ensuring timely payment.

12. Follow-up and Collections:

Follow-up and collections involve monitoring unpaid claims, aged accounts, and outstanding patient balances. Healthcare organizations need to proactively follow up on unpaid claims, communicate with patients regarding their outstanding balances, and implement effective collections strategies to maximize revenue recovery.

Each component of the revenue cycle plays a crucial role in the overall workflow. Efficient management of these components, from scheduling to collections, is vital for optimizing revenue, reducing claim denials, and ensuring financial stability. By understanding the workflow and interdependencies of these components, healthcare organizations can implement effective revenue cycle management strategies.

2.2 Key Terminologies in RCM:

Revenue cycle management (RCM) involves various industry-specific terminologies that are essential to understand for effective communication and implementation of revenue cycle processes. Here are key terminologies commonly used in RCM:

1. Clean Claim:

A clean claim refers to a claim that is complete, accurate, and error-free, meeting all the requirements for timely processing and payment by the insurance payer. Clean claims have a higher likelihood of being processed without delays or rejections.

2. Claim Denial:

A claim denial occurs when an insurance payer refuses to reimburse or pay for a submitted claim. Denials can happen due to various reasons, including missing information, coding errors, lack of medical necessity, eligibility issues, or contractual disputes. Effective denial management is crucial for resolving denials and maximizing revenue.

3. Accounts Receivable (AR):

Accounts Receivable refers to the outstanding balances owed to a healthcare organization for services rendered but not yet collected. AR typically includes insurance claims awaiting payment and patient balances. Monitoring and managing AR is important for optimizing cash flow and revenue collection.

4. Days in Accounts Receivable (DAR):

Days in Accounts Receivable represents the average number of days it takes for a healthcare organization to collect payments for services rendered. Lower DAR values indicate a more efficient revenue cycle, while higher values may suggest delays in reimbursement or inefficient collections processes.

5. Fee Schedule:

A fee schedule is a predetermined list of prices or reimbursement rates established by an insurance payer for specific healthcare services. It outlines the allowable amounts that will be paid for each service provided. Fee schedules vary across different payers and may impact reimbursement rates.

6. Explanation of Benefits (EOB):

An Explanation of Benefits is a document provided by an insurance payer to a patient or healthcare provider, detailing the services rendered, the amount billed, the amount paid, and any remaining patient responsibilities. EOBs provide valuable information for reconciling payments and resolving billing inquiries.

7. Remittance Advice (RA):

A Remittance Advice is a communication document sent by an insurance payer to a healthcare provider, summarizing the payment details for processed claims. RAs include information on the services paid, payment amounts, adjustments, denials, and reasons for any discrepancies.

8. Medical Coding:

Medical coding is the process of translating healthcare procedures, diagnoses, and services into standardized codes. Common coding systems include Current Procedural Terminology (CPT) for procedures and services and International Classification of Diseases (ICD) for diagnoses. Accurate coding is vital for proper billing, claims submission, and reimbursement.

9. Charge Description Master (CDM):

The Charge Description Master, also known as the chargemaster, is a comprehensive listing of healthcare services provided by a healthcare organization, along with their associated prices or charge amounts. The CDM serves as the basis for charge capture, billing, and revenue calculations.

10. Electronic Data Interchange (EDI):

Electronic Data Interchange is the electronic exchange of healthcare information between different entities, such as healthcare providers, insurance companies, and clearinghouses. EDI formats, such as HIPAA-compliant X12 standards, facilitate the seamless transmission of claims, remittance advice, and other revenue cycle-related data.

Understanding these key terminologies helps healthcare professionals navigate the complexities of revenue cycle management and facilitates effective communication with stakeholders involved in the revenue cycle process.

2.3 Understanding Payer Types and Reimbursement Models:

In revenue cycle management (RCM), it is crucial to understand the different payer types and reimbursement models that impact the billing and reimbursement processes. Let's explore the common payer types and reimbursement models in healthcare:

1. Private Insurance Payers:

Private insurance payers include commercial health insurance companies that individuals or employers purchase to provide healthcare coverage. These payers typically have their own policies, coverage criteria, and reimbursement rates. Private insurance payers may have varying networks of healthcare providers, and reimbursement rates are often negotiated through contracts.

2. Government Payers:

Government payers include federal and state-funded programs that provide healthcare coverage to eligible individuals. The two primary government payers in the United States are:

a. Medicare: Medicare is a federal health insurance program primarily for individuals aged 65 and older, certain younger individuals with disabilities, and individuals with end-stage renal disease. Medicare has different parts, such as Part A (hospital insurance), Part B (medical insurance), Part C (Medicare Advantage plans), and Part D (prescription drug coverage).

b. Medicaid: Medicaid is a joint federal and state program that provides healthcare coverage to low-income individuals and families. Medicaid eligibility and coverage criteria vary by state, and reimbursement rates are typically lower than those of private payers.

3. Managed Care Organizations (MCOs):

Managed Care Organizations are entities that contract with payers, such as private insurance companies or government programs, to manage healthcare services and control costs. MCOs employ various models, including Health Maintenance Organizations (HMOs), Preferred Provider Organizations (PPOs), and Accountable Care Organizations (ACOs). These models involve negotiated contracts and specific provider networks, often requiring prior authorizations and utilization management for services.

4. Self-Funded Employer Plans:

Some employers self-fund their employee healthcare plans, meaning they assume the financial risk for providing healthcare benefits. In these plans, employers may contract with third-party administrators (TPAs) for claims processing and administrative functions. Reimbursement rates and policies are determined by the employer's plan.

5. Value-Based Reimbursement Models:

Value-based reimbursement models aim to incentivize quality care outcomes rather than paying solely based on services rendered. These models include:

a. Pay-for-Performance (P4P): Providers receive additional reimbursement or incentives based on achieving predetermined quality measures or performance metrics.

b. Bundled Payments: Reimbursement is provided for an entire episode of care rather than individual services. Providers are responsible for managing costs and quality across the entire care continuum.

c. Accountable Care Organizations (ACOs): ACOs are groups of healthcare providers that voluntarily come together to coordinate care for a defined patient population. Providers are financially rewarded for improving quality and reducing costs.

Understanding the various payer types and reimbursement models is crucial for healthcare organizations to navigate billing and reimbursement processes effectively. It helps ensure accurate claims submission, adherence to payer-specific guidelines, negotiation of favorable contracts, and optimization of revenue cycle performance.

Exercise 2: Revenue Cycle Basics

1. Revenue Cycle Components and Workflow

Question 1: List the key components of the revenue cycle.

Answer: The key components of the revenue cycle include:

- Patient registration and demographic data collection

- Insurance verification and eligibility checking

- Patient financial responsibility and estimation

- Scheduling and patient access management

- Medical coding and documentation

- Charge capture and reimbursement

- Claims submission and adjudication

- Denial management and appeals

- Insurance follow-up and accounts receivable management

- Patient billing and collections

Question 2: Describe the typical workflow of the revenue cycle.

Answer: The typical workflow of the revenue cycle involves the following steps:

1. Patient Registration: Collecting patient demographic information, insurance details, and consent forms.

2. Insurance Verification and Eligibility: Verifying insurance coverage and eligibility to ensure the services will be covered.

3. Patient Financial Responsibility: Estimating and communicating the patient's financial responsibility, including copayments, deductibles, and coinsurance.

4. Scheduling and Patient Access: Managing appointments, ensuring efficient patient flow, and addressing any access-related issues.

5. Medical Coding and Documentation: Assigning appropriate codes to procedures and diagnoses based on the medical documentation.

6. Charge Capture: Capturing charges for services rendered accurately and completely.

7. Reimbursement: Submitting claims to payers, including insurance companies or government programs, for reimbursement.

8. Claims Adjudication: Payers review and process claims, determining the payment amount based on contractual agreements, coverage policies, and medical necessity.

9. Denial Management and Appeals: Addressing claim denials, identifying the root causes, and initiating appeals when necessary.

10. Insurance Follow-Up and Accounts Receivable Management: Monitoring unpaid claims, communicating with payers, and taking necessary actions to ensure timely reimbursement.

11. Patient Billing and Collections: Generating patient bills, explaining charges, facilitating payment options, and managing collections.

2. Key Terminologies in RCM

Question 1: Define the following key terminologies in revenue cycle management:

a) CPT Codes

b) ICD Codes

c) EOB

Answer:

a) CPT Codes: Current Procedural Terminology (CPT) codes are standardized codes used to describe medical procedures and services provided by healthcare professionals. These codes are published by the American Medical Association (AMA) and are essential for accurate billing and claims submission.

b) ICD Codes: International Classification of Diseases (ICD) codes are alphanumeric codes used to classify and code diagnoses, symptoms, and procedures in healthcare. These codes provide a standardized way to document and report medical conditions, enabling accurate billing, data analysis, and research.

c) EOB: Explanation of Benefits (EOB) is a document sent by insurance companies to patients and providers that explains the outcome of a claim. It provides details about the services covered, payment made, patient responsibility, and any adjustments or denials.

3. Understanding Payer Types and Reimbursement Models

Question 1: Explain the difference between primary and secondary payers.

Answer: Primary and secondary payers refer to the order in which insurance coverage is applied when multiple insurance plans are involved:

- Primary Payer: The primary payer is the insurance plan that has the primary responsibility for paying healthcare claims. It is typically the insurance plan of the individual or the policyholder. The primary payer is billed first for services rendered, and once the claim is processed, the secondary payer is billed for any remaining balance.

- Secondary Payer: The secondary payer is the insurance plan that covers the remaining balance after the primary payer has processed the claim. It is usually another insurance plan, such as a spouse's insurance or a supplemental insurance plan. The secondary payer reimburses the provider for the additional costs not covered by the primary payer.

Question 2: Describe the fee-for-service and value-based reimbursement models.

Answer:

- Fee-for-Service (FFS) Reimbursement Model: In the fee-for-service model, healthcare providers are reimbursed based on the specific services or procedures they provide. Each service is assigned a predetermined fee or reimbursement rate. Providers submit claims for each service rendered, and payment is made based on the agreed-upon fee schedule or the negotiated rate with the payer.

- Value-Based Reimbursement Model: In the value-based reimbursement model, reimbursement is tied to the quality and outcomes of care rather than the quantity of services provided. Providers are incentivized to deliver high-quality, cost-effective care by meeting certain performance metrics and achieving predefined outcomes. This model promotes value, efficiency, and patient-centered care delivery.

These exercises provide an opportunity to reinforce the knowledge gained from the chapter on Revenue Cycle Basics. The questions assess understanding and reinforce key concepts related to the components and workflow of the revenue cycle, key terminologies in RCM (CPT codes, ICD codes, EOB), and understanding primary and secondary payers, as well as fee-for-service and value-based reimbursement models.

3. Revenue Cycle Management Planning

3.1 Setting RCM Goals and Objectives:

Setting clear goals and objectives is a crucial step in effective revenue cycle management (RCM) planning. Well-defined goals provide direction, focus, and measurable targets to guide RCM efforts. When setting RCM goals and objectives, consider the following:

1. Financial Goals:

Identify financial goals that align with the overall financial objectives of the healthcare organization. Examples of financial goals include increasing revenue collections, reducing days in accounts receivable (DAR), improving cash flow, minimizing bad debt, and optimizing net revenue.

2. Operational Goals:

Define operational goals that improve the efficiency and effectiveness of revenue cycle processes. Examples of operational goals include reducing claim denials, streamlining workflow and process automation, enhancing coding accuracy, improving charge capture, and minimizing billing errors.

3. Performance Goals:

Establish performance goals that measure the effectiveness of revenue cycle performance. Key performance indicators (KPIs) help monitor and evaluate progress. Examples of performance goals include achieving a target clean claim rate, reducing claim rejection rates, improving first-pass resolution rates, and decreasing the percentage of accounts in the 90+ days category.

4. Patient Satisfaction Goals:

Consider patient satisfaction goals as an integral part of RCM planning. Happy and satisfied patients are more likely to fulfill their financial responsibilities and recommend the healthcare organization to others. Patient satisfaction goals may involve improving billing transparency, enhancing customer service, and simplifying the payment process.

5. Compliance and Regulatory Goals:

Ensure that compliance and regulatory goals are incorporated into RCM planning. Compliance with regulations such as HIPAA, coding guidelines, and payer-specific policies is crucial. Goals may include maintaining a high level of compliance, conducting regular audits, and staying updated with changing regulations.

6. Technology and Process Improvement Goals:

Identify goals related to leveraging technology and process improvement initiatives. Examples include implementing or upgrading revenue cycle management systems, enhancing electronic health record (EHR) integration, optimizing automation and artificial intelligence tools, and streamlining data analytics for better decision-making.

7. Staff Training and Development Goals:

Recognize the importance of staff training and development in achieving RCM objectives. Goals may include providing ongoing training programs on coding and billing regulations, enhancing communication and customer service skills, and fostering a culture of continuous improvement.

8. Collaboration and Communication Goals:

Emphasize goals that foster collaboration and effective communication among revenue cycle team members, healthcare providers, and other stakeholders. This ensures coordination, transparency, and shared accountability in revenue cycle processes.

When setting RCM goals and objectives, ensure they are specific, measurable, achievable, relevant, and time-bound (SMART). Break down long-term goals into short-term objectives and define key milestones and timelines for monitoring progress.

Regularly assess and reassess RCM goals to ensure they remain aligned with evolving organizational priorities, industry changes, and emerging trends. Engage stakeholders across the organization to gain their input and foster buy-in for RCM goals and objectives.

Setting clear RCM goals and objectives provides a roadmap for effective planning, resource allocation, and performance measurement. It establishes a framework for continuous improvement and guides the implementation of strategies to optimize the revenue cycle.

3.2 Assessing Organizational Readiness for RCM:

Assessing organizational readiness for revenue cycle management (RCM) is crucial before implementing any RCM initiatives. It involves evaluating various aspects of the organization to determine its preparedness for effective RCM implementation. Here are key factors to consider when assessing organizational readiness:

1. Leadership Support and Commitment:

Evaluate the level of support and commitment from organizational leadership towards RCM initiatives. Leadership buy-in is essential for allocating resources, promoting a culture of accountability, and driving necessary changes within the organization.

2. Organizational Culture:

Assess the existing organizational culture to determine if it is conducive to RCM success. A culture that values transparency, collaboration, continuous improvement, and a focus on financial performance fosters an environment that supports effective RCM practices.

3. Staff Competency and Training:

Evaluate the knowledge, skills, and expertise of the revenue cycle team and other staff involved in RCM processes. Assess their understanding of coding, billing regulations, payer guidelines, and the use of RCM software. Identify training needs and develop a plan to enhance staff competency.

4. Technology Infrastructure:

Evaluate the organization's technology infrastructure, including the electronic health record (EHR) system, billing and coding software, and other RCM tools. Assess the compatibility, functionality, and integration capabilities of existing systems to support efficient revenue cycle processes.

5. Data Management and Analytics:

Assess the organization's ability to capture, manage, and analyze revenue cycle data. Evaluate the availability and accuracy of data related to key performance indicators (KPIs) such as clean claim rates, denial rates, days in accounts receivable, and collections. Identify any gaps in data collection and reporting processes.

6. Workflow and Process Evaluation:

Evaluate current revenue cycle workflows and processes. Identify bottlenecks, inefficiencies, and areas of potential improvement. Assess the effectiveness of existing policies and procedures, and determine if they align with industry best practices and regulatory requirements.

7. Financial and Resource Allocation:

Assess the organization's financial resources allocated to RCM. Evaluate if sufficient resources are available to invest in technology, staff training, process improvement initiatives, and any necessary external expertise.

8. Regulatory Compliance:

Evaluate the organization's compliance with regulatory requirements and industry standards. Assess the implementation of policies and procedures related to patient data privacy (HIPAA), coding guidelines, claim submission, and reimbursement regulations.

9. Payer and Contract Management:

Assess the organization's ability to manage payer relationships and contracts effectively. Evaluate the processes for verifying insurance eligibility, negotiating contracts, and monitoring reimbursement rates. Identify any challenges or gaps in payer management.

10. Stakeholder Engagement:

Assess the engagement and collaboration of stakeholders involved in the revenue cycle, such as healthcare providers, administrators, finance staff, and patients. Evaluate their understanding of RCM goals, their willingness to adapt to changes, and their involvement in process improvement initiatives.

Based on the assessment, identify areas of strength and areas that require improvement. Develop an action plan to address any gaps, allocate necessary resources, and prioritize initiatives for successful RCM implementation.

Regular reassessment of organizational readiness is essential, considering that RCM is an ongoing process influenced by evolving industry dynamics, technology advancements, and regulatory changes. Continuously monitoring organizational readiness ensures the organization remains prepared to adapt and optimize revenue cycle management practices.

Developing a well-defined implementation strategy is essential for successful revenue cycle management (RCM) adoption within an organization. An effective strategy outlines the necessary steps, timelines, and resources required to implement RCM initiatives. Here are key considerations when developing an RCM implementation strategy:

1. Define RCM Objectives:

Clearly articulate the specific objectives and goals of the RCM implementation. Align these objectives with the overall organizational goals, financial targets, and performance improvement initiatives. Ensure that the objectives are specific, measurable, achievable, relevant, and time-bound (SMART).

2. Establish an Implementation Team:

Assemble a multidisciplinary team comprising representatives from finance, revenue cycle, IT, clinical departments, and administration. This team will oversee the RCM implementation, coordinate activities, and ensure effective communication and collaboration across departments.

3. Conduct Gap Analysis:

Perform a comprehensive gap analysis to identify areas of improvement in the existing revenue cycle processes. Assess the gaps in terms of technology, workflow, staff competency, policies, and compliance. This analysis will serve as the foundation for developing strategies to address identified gaps.

4. Prioritize Initiatives:

Prioritize the identified gaps and initiatives based on their impact, urgency, and feasibility. Determine which initiatives will deliver the most significant improvement in revenue cycle performance. Consider both short-term quick wins and long-term strategic initiatives in the prioritization process.

5. Develop Action Plans:

For each prioritized initiative, develop detailed action plans outlining the steps, resources, and timelines required for implementation. Assign responsibilities to team members and ensure accountability for each action item. Break down larger initiatives into smaller manageable tasks to facilitate implementation and progress tracking.

6. Allocate Resources:

Determine the resources needed to support the RCM implementation. This includes financial resources for technology investments, staff training, process improvement initiatives, and any external expertise required. Ensure that the necessary resources are allocated to support the implementation plan.

7. Technology Considerations:

Assess the technology infrastructure required to support the RCM initiatives. Evaluate if existing systems can meet the desired objectives or if new technology solutions need to be acquired or integrated. Consider the implementation timeline, system compatibility, data migration, and user training when planning technology-related initiatives.

8. Training and Change Management:

Develop a comprehensive training plan to enhance staff competency and ensure a smooth transition to new processes and systems. Provide training on coding and documentation guidelines, RCM software, workflow changes, and compliance requirements. Implement change management strategies to address staff resistance and facilitate adoption.

9. Communication and Stakeholder Engagement:

Develop a communication plan to engage stakeholders throughout the RCM implementation. Regularly communicate the progress, benefits, and impact of the initiatives to staff, healthcare providers, and administrators. Seek input and feedback from stakeholders to ensure their involvement and support.

10. Performance Monitoring and Evaluation:

Establish performance monitoring mechanisms to track the progress and outcomes of the RCM initiatives. Define key performance indicators (KPIs) aligned with the RCM objectives and establish regular reporting and review cycles. Continuously evaluate the effectiveness of the implementation strategy and make adjustments as needed.

11. Continuous Improvement:

Emphasize the importance of continuous improvement in RCM. Encourage a culture of ongoing assessment, feedback, and refinement of processes. Engage staff in identifying opportunities for improvement, implementing best practices, and sharing lessons learned.

By developing a comprehensive RCM implementation strategy, organizations can ensure a systematic and successful adoption of revenue cycle management practices. The strategy provides a roadmap for achieving RCM objectives, optimizing financial performance, and enhancing operational efficiency.

Implementing revenue cycle management (RCM) initiatives often involves significant changes to processes, systems, and roles within an organization. Effective change management is essential to ensure successful RCM adoption and minimize resistance from staff. Here are key considerations for managing change in RCM:

1. Develop a Change Management Plan:

Create a structured change management plan that outlines the approach, activities, and timelines for managing the RCM implementation. Include strategies for communication, stakeholder engagement, training, and addressing resistance. The plan should align with the overall RCM implementation strategy.

2. Communicate the Need for Change:

Clearly communicate the reasons behind the RCM initiatives, emphasizing the benefits and positive impact on staff and the organization as a whole. Explain how RCM will improve revenue performance, streamline processes, enhance patient satisfaction, and support the organization's strategic goals.

3. Engage Stakeholders:

Involve key stakeholders, such as revenue cycle staff, healthcare providers, and administrative personnel, throughout the RCM implementation process. Seek their input, address their concerns, and involve them in decision-making. Create opportunities for collaboration, feedback, and ownership of the changes.

4. Create a Shared Vision:

Develop a shared vision for the RCM implementation, emphasizing the benefits and outcomes that the organization aims to achieve. Align the vision with the overall organizational goals and values. Communicate the vision consistently and reinforce it throughout the implementation process.

5. Provide Training and Support:

Offer comprehensive training programs to ensure that staff members have the necessary knowledge and skills to adapt to the changes. Provide training on new processes, technology systems, coding guidelines, and any other relevant areas. Offer ongoing support and resources to assist staff during the transition.

6. Address Resistance:

Anticipate and address resistance to change by identifying potential challenges and concerns. Engage in open and honest communication to address fears, misconceptions, and uncertainties. Create a safe space for staff to express their concerns and provide opportunities for dialogue and problem-solving.

7. Empower Change Champions:

Identify change champions within the organization who can serve as advocates for RCM initiatives. These individuals can help drive the change, provide peer support, and share success stories. Empower them with the necessary resources and authority to support the implementation.

8. Monitor and Celebrate Progress:

Regularly monitor the progress of the RCM implementation and celebrate milestones and successes along the way. Recognize and appreciate staff efforts and achievements. Provide feedback on the positive impact of the changes to motivate and sustain momentum.

9. Continuously Evaluate and Adjust:

Continuously evaluate the effectiveness of the change management strategies and make adjustments as needed. Solicit feedback from staff and stakeholders to identify areas for improvement. Learn from challenges and successes to refine the change management approach.

10. Sustain the Change:

Ensure that the changes implemented through RCM initiatives become embedded in the organization's culture and practices. Reinforce the new processes, provide ongoing training and support, and incorporate RCM practices into performance evaluations and quality improvement initiatives.

By implementing effective change management strategies, organizations can foster a positive and supportive environment for RCM adoption. This approach helps mitigate resistance, engage stakeholders, and increase the likelihood of successful RCM implementation and long-term sustainability.

Exercise 3: Revenue Cycle Management Planning

1. Setting RCM Goals and Objectives

Question 1: Why is it important for healthcare organizations to set specific goals and objectives for revenue cycle management (RCM)?

Answer: Setting specific goals and objectives for RCM is important for healthcare organizations because:

- It provides a clear direction: Goals and objectives help guide the organization's efforts and establish a clear direction for RCM initiatives.

- It enhances focus and alignment: Having specific goals and objectives ensures that everyone within the organization is aligned and focused on the same objectives, facilitating effective teamwork and collaboration.

- It promotes accountability: Clear goals and objectives enable accountability for performance and outcomes, allowing organizations to measure progress and hold individuals and teams responsible.

- It supports continuous improvement: Goals and objectives provide a basis for evaluating RCM processes and identifying areas for improvement, leading to enhanced efficiency and effectiveness.

- It drives strategic decision-making: Well-defined goals and objectives inform strategic decision-making by aligning RCM initiatives with broader organizational goals and priorities.

Question 2: Provide examples of specific goals and objectives that a healthcare organization may set for RCM.

Answer: Examples of specific goals and objectives for RCM may include:

- Increase clean claim rate by 10% within six months.

- Reduce claim denials by 20% within one year.

- Improve patient collections by implementing a new patient-friendly billing system.

- Enhance coding accuracy and achieve a coding accuracy rate of 95%.

- Streamline the prior authorization process to reduce delays and improve revenue cycle efficiency.

- Implement automated RCM software to optimize billing and claims management processes.

- Enhance staff training and education on RCM best practices to improve overall performance.

2. Assessing Organizational Readiness for RCM

Question 1: Why is it important for healthcare organizations to assess their readiness before implementing revenue cycle management (RCM) initiatives?

Answer: Assessing organizational readiness is important before implementing RCM initiatives because:

- It helps identify strengths and weaknesses: Assessing readiness enables organizations to identify their existing capabilities and areas that require improvement. It helps understand the organization's readiness to effectively implement and manage RCM initiatives.

- It aids in resource allocation: By assessing readiness, organizations can determine the resources needed for successful RCM implementation, including staffing, technology, training, and financial resources.

- It facilitates strategic planning: An assessment of readiness provides insights that support strategic planning for RCM initiatives. It helps prioritize areas of focus, establish realistic timelines, and set achievable goals.

- It mitigates risks: Assessing readiness helps organizations identify potential risks and challenges associated with RCM implementation. It allows proactive risk management and the development of mitigation strategies.

- It promotes stakeholder engagement: Assessing readiness involves engaging stakeholders, such as staff members, providers, and administrators, in the process. Their input and involvement contribute to a more effective and successful implementation.

Question 2: What are some key areas that healthcare organizations should assess when evaluating their readiness for RCM implementation?

Answer: Healthcare organizations should assess the following key areas when evaluating their readiness for RCM implementation:

- Leadership support and commitment to RCM initiatives.

- Adequacy of staffing and resources for RCM implementation.

- Current technology infrastructure and systems to support RCM processes.

- Knowledge and competency levels of staff in RCM best practices.

- Existing workflows and processes related to revenue cycle management.

- Availability and quality of data for reporting and analytics in RCM.

- Organizational culture and readiness for change management.

3. Developing an RCM Implementation Strategy

Question 1: Why is it important for healthcare organizations to develop a comprehensive implementation strategy for revenue cycle management (RCM)?

Answer: Developing a comprehensive implementation strategy for RCM is important for healthcare organizations because:

- It provides a roadmap: An implementation strategy outlines the step-by-step approach to be followed during the RCM implementation process. It serves as a roadmap for organizations, ensuring a systematic and organized approach to implementation.

- It aligns stakeholders: An implementation strategy helps align stakeholders by clearly communicating the goals, objectives, and timelines of the RCM initiative. It ensures that all individuals and teams involved are working towards a common vision.

- It facilitates resource allocation: A well-developed implementation strategy helps organizations allocate the necessary resources, including human, financial, and technological resources, for successful RCM implementation.

- It minimizes disruptions: An implementation strategy considers potential risks and challenges and incorporates mitigation strategies. This helps minimize disruptions and ensures smooth implementation while maintaining business continuity.

- It promotes accountability and evaluation: A comprehensive strategy defines milestones and performance metrics, enabling organizations to track progress, measure outcomes, and hold individuals and teams accountable for their roles in the implementation process.

Question 2: What are the key components that should be included in an RCM implementation strategy?

Answer: Key components that should be included in an RCM implementation strategy are:

- Clear objectives and goals: Define specific objectives and goals that the organization aims to achieve through the implementation of RCM initiatives.

- Timeline and milestones: Establish a realistic timeline with specific milestones to track progress and ensure timely completion of each phase of the implementation process.

- Resource allocation: Identify the necessary resources, including financial, technological, and human resources, and allocate them appropriately to support the implementation.

- Change management plan: Develop a change management plan to address the cultural and organizational changes that may arise during the implementation process. It should include strategies for communication, training, and stakeholder engagement.

- Performance metrics and evaluation: Define key performance indicators (KPIs) and metrics to assess the success and effectiveness of the implemented RCM initiatives. Establish mechanisms for ongoing evaluation and continuous improvement.

- Risk assessment and mitigation: Identify potential risks and challenges that may arise during the implementation and develop strategies to mitigate them. This ensures proactive risk management and minimizes disruptions.

- Communication and stakeholder engagement: Develop a comprehensive communication plan to ensure effective communication with stakeholders at all levels, including staff, providers, and leadership.

4. Change Management in RCM

Question 1: Why is change management important in the context of revenue cycle management (RCM) implementation?

Answer: Change management is important in the context of RCM implementation because:

- Resistance to change: Change can be met with resistance from staff members who may be accustomed to existing processes. Effective change management helps address resistance, mitigate fears, and gain buy-in from individuals and teams involved in RCM implementation.

- Adoption and engagement: Change management strategies foster adoption and engagement by ensuring that individuals understand the benefits and rationale behind RCM initiatives. It encourages active participation and involvement in the implementation process.

- Minimizing disruptions: RCM implementation involves changes in workflows, processes, and technology systems. Change management helps minimize disruptions by providing support, training, and clear communication to ensure a smooth transition.

- Sustainability: Change management promotes the sustainability of RCM initiatives by embedding the new processes and practices into the organizational culture. It ensures that the changes are not temporary but become an integral part of daily operations.

- Maximizing benefits: Effective change management ensures that the intended benefits and outcomes of RCM implementation are achieved. It supports the realization of performance improvements, cost savings, and enhanced revenue cycle efficiency.

Question 2: What are some strategies that healthcare organizations can employ to manage change effectively during RCM implementation?

Answer: Healthcare organizations can employ the following strategies to manage change effectively during RCM implementation:

- Leadership involvement and support: Engage leaders who are visible advocates for RCM initiatives and actively participate in the change process. Their support and involvement set the tone for the rest of the organization.

- Clear communication: Develop a communication plan that includes regular and transparent communication about the goals, benefits, and progress of RCM implementation. Provide forums for staff to ask questions, share concerns, and provide feedback.

- Training and education: Provide comprehensive training and education to ensure that staff members understand the new processes, technologies, and their roles in the RCM implementation. Offer ongoing support and resources to address skill gaps and facilitate a smooth transition.

- Stakeholder engagement: Involve stakeholders from various levels and departments in the planning and decision-making processes. Seek their input, address their concerns, and incorporate their perspectives to increase buy-in and ownership.

- Pilot programs and phased approach: Implement RCM initiatives in pilot programs or phases, allowing for testing, feedback, and adjustments before full-scale implementation. This approach reduces the risk of disruption and provides opportunities for continuous improvement.

- Celebrate successes: Recognize and celebrate achievements and milestones throughout the RCM implementation journey. This helps maintain motivation and momentum and reinforces the positive impact of the changes.

These exercises provide an opportunity to reinforce the knowledge gained from the chapter on Revenue Cycle Management Planning. The questions assess understanding and reinforce key concepts related to setting goals and objectives, assessing organizational readiness, developing an implementation strategy, and managing change during RCM implementation.

4. Patient Registration and Pre-Service Revenue Cycle

4.1 Patient Pre-Registration and Demographic Data Collection:

The first step in the revenue cycle is patient registration, which involves collecting accurate and comprehensive demographic and insurance information. Proper patient pre-registration and demographic data collection are crucial for ensuring a smooth revenue cycle process. Let's explore the key considerations for patient pre-registration and demographic data collection:

1. Pre-Registration Process:

Pre-registration involves collecting patient information before their scheduled appointment or visit. This can be done through various channels, including online portals, phone calls, or in-person interactions. The pre-registration process helps streamline the patient check-in process, reducing wait times and ensuring a more efficient revenue cycle.

2. Demographic Data Collection:

Collecting accurate demographic information is essential for identifying patients, verifying insurance coverage, and establishing the financial account. Demographic data typically include:

a. Personal Information: Gather the patient's full name, date of birth, gender, address, phone number, and email address. Ensure that the information is recorded accurately and without errors.

b. Identification Documents: Collect identification documents, such as a driver's license or government-issued ID, to verify the patient's identity.

c. Insurance Information: Obtain the patient's insurance details, including the insurance company name, policy number, group number, and primary insured's information. Verify the insurance coverage and eligibility to determine the patient's financial responsibility.

d. Emergency Contact Details: Request emergency contact information, including the name, relationship, and contact number of a person to reach in case of an emergency.

e. Medical History: Capture relevant medical history information, such as previous diagnoses, allergies, medications, and past surgical procedures. This data helps healthcare providers deliver appropriate care and supports accurate coding and documentation.

f. Consent and Privacy Forms: Ensure that patients complete necessary consent forms, such as HIPAA authorization and release of information forms. Inform patients about their rights regarding the use and disclosure of their protected health information (PHI).

3. Verification of Demographic Information:

Verify the accuracy of the demographic information provided by patients. Use electronic verification tools or contact patients directly to validate their personal and insurance information. This step helps prevent claim denials and reduces billing errors.

4. Patient Communication:

Maintain clear and open communication with patients during the pre-registration process. Explain the importance of accurate information and how it impacts billing and reimbursement. Address any questions or concerns they may have regarding insurance coverage, financial responsibilities, or privacy rights.

5. Data Security and Privacy:

Ensure compliance with HIPAA regulations and maintain strict data security and privacy protocols. Safeguard patient information, both in physical and electronic formats, to protect against unauthorized access or breaches.

6. Technology and Automation:

Utilize electronic systems and patient portals to streamline the pre-registration process. Offer online pre-registration options that allow patients to enter their information directly into the system. Automated verification tools can help validate insurance eligibility and streamline data entry.

7. Staff Training:

Train registration staff on proper data collection techniques, privacy regulations, and effective patient communication. Provide ongoing training to keep staff updated on changes in insurance requirements, coding guidelines, and best practices in patient pre-registration.

Accurate patient pre-registration and demographic data collection are vital for setting the foundation of a successful revenue cycle. By implementing efficient processes, leveraging technology, and ensuring staff competency, healthcare organizations can streamline the registration process, reduce errors, and facilitate a seamless revenue cycle workflow.

4.2 Insurance Verification and Eligibility Checking:

Insurance verification and eligibility checking are critical components of the revenue cycle process. Verifying insurance coverage and confirming patient eligibility help ensure accurate billing, reduce claim denials, and facilitate timely reimbursement. Here are key considerations for insurance verification and eligibility checking:

1. Collect Insurance Information:

Obtain the patient's insurance details during the registration process, including the insurance company name, policy number, group number, and primary insured's information. Ensure that the information is accurately recorded and entered into the system.

2. Insurance Company Contact:

Contact the patient's insurance company to verify coverage and eligibility. This can be done through various channels, such as phone calls, online portals, or electronic data interchange (EDI) transactions. Use the designated contact methods provided by the insurance company for efficient communication.

3. Insurance Coverage Verification:

Confirm the patient's insurance coverage for the specific services to be rendered. Verify the effective dates of coverage, the type of plan (e.g., HMO, PPO), and any limitations or exclusions that may impact reimbursement. Ensure that the services to be provided are covered under the patient's insurance plan.

4. Co-Payments, Deductibles, and Co-Insurance:

Determine the patient's financial responsibilities, including co-payments, deductibles, and co-insurance amounts. Communicate this information to the patient before the services are rendered, allowing them to understand their financial obligations.

5. Eligibility Checking:

Check the patient's eligibility for the services to be provided. Verify that the patient's insurance plan covers the specific procedures, treatments, or tests scheduled. Confirm any pre-authorization requirements or additional documentation needed for claim submission.

6. Online Verification Tools:

Utilize online verification tools and electronic data interchange (EDI) transactions to streamline the eligibility checking process. Many insurance companies offer online portals or real-time eligibility verification systems that provide instant access to patient eligibility and coverage details.

7. Document Verification:

Maintain accurate documentation of the verification process, including the date, time, and details of communication with the insurance company. Retain records of the eligibility verification for reference and potential audits.

8. Follow-Up and Updates:

Regularly follow up with insurance companies to ensure continued eligibility throughout the patient's treatment or care plan. Update the patient's insurance information as necessary, especially if there are changes in coverage, policy numbers, or primary insured details.

9. Communication with Patients:

Clearly communicate the results of insurance verification and eligibility checking to patients. Inform them about any financial responsibilities, including co-payments, deductibles, or co-insurance amounts they need to fulfill. Provide them with a breakdown of the estimated costs and offer guidance on financial assistance programs, if applicable.

10. Compliance with Insurance Requirements:

Adhere to the specific requirements and guidelines set by insurance companies. Familiarize yourself with the insurer's policies regarding pre-authorization, medical necessity, and documentation. Ensure that the provided services meet the insurer's guidelines to minimize claim denials.

Effective insurance verification and eligibility checking processes contribute to accurate billing, reduced claim denials, and improved revenue cycle performance. By leveraging technology, maintaining clear communication with patients, and adhering to insurance requirements, healthcare organizations can streamline the revenue cycle and optimize reimbursement.

Patient financial responsibility and estimation play a crucial role in revenue cycle management. Providing patients with accurate and transparent information about their financial obligations helps promote financial clarity, improve collections, and enhance patient satisfaction. Here are key considerations for managing patient financial responsibility and estimation:

1. Insurance Coverage Review:

Review the patient's insurance coverage to determine the extent of their financial responsibility. Understand the insurance plan's co-payment, deductible, and co-insurance requirements. Familiarize yourself with any limitations, exclusions, or non-covered services that may impact the patient's financial obligations.

2. Educate Patients about Insurance Benefits:

Educate patients on their insurance benefits, including coverage details and limitations. Clearly explain concepts such as co-payments, deductibles, and co-insurance, ensuring that patients understand their financial responsibilities and how they affect their out-of-pocket costs.

3. Financial Counseling:

Offer financial counseling services to patients to help them navigate the complexities of insurance coverage and healthcare costs. Provide guidance on understanding insurance policies, estimating costs, and exploring financial assistance options.

4. Transparent Cost Estimation:

Provide patients with transparent and accurate cost estimates for the services they will receive. Use pricing information, fee schedules, and insurance contract terms to calculate the patient's expected out-of-pocket costs. Explain the estimation methodology and any assumptions made.

5. Cost Estimation Tools:

Leverage cost estimation tools or software that can integrate with billing systems and insurance data to generate real-time cost estimates. These tools consider factors such as insurance coverage, deductibles, and co-insurance rates to provide accurate estimates to patients.

6. Communication of Financial Estimates:

Clearly communicate the estimated costs to patients, ensuring they are aware of their financial responsibility before receiving services. Provide a breakdown of the estimated charges, including the expected insurance coverage and the patient's portion. Offer multiple channels for communication, such as in-person discussions, written estimates, or online portals.

7. Point-of-Service Collections:

Implement point-of-service (POS) collections processes to collect patient financial obligations at the time of service. Train staff to communicate with patients about their financial responsibility, explain payment options, and facilitate prompt collections. Offer convenient payment methods, such as credit cards, electronic transfers, or payment plans, to improve collections.

8. Financial Assistance Programs:

Assess and inform patients about available financial assistance programs, such as charity care or sliding scale fee programs. Provide guidance on the application process and eligibility criteria, ensuring that patients in need have access to financial support.

9. Clear Billing Statements:

Generate clear and itemized billing statements that outline the services provided, insurance adjustments, and the patient's financial responsibility. Ensure that the billing statements are easy to understand and include contact information for billing inquiries or payment arrangements.

10. Patient Follow-Up:

Follow up with patients regarding outstanding balances or unresolved billing inquiries. Implement effective processes to address patient concerns, provide necessary explanations, and resolve any billing disputes promptly. Maintain open lines of communication to build trust and maintain positive patient-provider relationships.

11. Compliance with Billing Regulations:

Adhere to billing regulations, such as those outlined by the Health Insurance Portability and Accountability Act (HIPAA) and the Fair Debt Collection Practices Act (FDCPA). Ensure that patient financial information is protected and billing practices are in compliance with legal requirements.

Effectively managing patient financial responsibility and estimation promotes transparency, patient satisfaction, and optimized revenue cycle outcomes. By implementing clear communication, accurate estimation methods, and appropriate financial counseling, healthcare organizations can improve collections, minimize billing disputes, and foster positive patient experiences.

1. Patient Pre-Registration and Demographic Data Collection

Question 1: Why is patient pre-registration important in the revenue cycle management (RCM) process?

Answer: Patient pre-registration is important in the RCM process because:

- It ensures accurate and complete patient demographic information, which is essential for billing and claims submission.

- It streamlines the registration process by collecting necessary information in advance, reducing wait times for patients.

- It helps verify insurance coverage and eligibility before the patient's visit, allowing for proactive financial planning and minimizing payment-related issues.

- It improves patient satisfaction by reducing paperwork and providing a more efficient and personalized registration experience.

Question 2: What are the key components of patient pre-registration and demographic data collection?

Answer: The key components of patient pre-registration and demographic data collection include:

- Collecting patient's personal information (name, address, contact details, etc.)

- Verifying patient identification and ensuring accuracy of data entry

- Gathering insurance information, including policy details and payer information

- Capturing demographic data such as date of birth, gender, and social security number

- Obtaining necessary consents and signatures, such as privacy policies and financial responsibility agreements

- Recording relevant medical history and any known allergies or conditions

2. Insurance Verification and Eligibility Checking

Question 1: Why is insurance verification and eligibility checking important in the revenue cycle management (RCM) process?

Answer: Insurance verification and eligibility checking are important in the RCM process because:

- They ensure that the patient's insurance coverage is valid and active before services are rendered, reducing the risk of claim denials and payment delays.

- They help determine the patient's financial responsibility, including copayments, deductibles, and coinsurance, enabling accurate estimation of costs and facilitating upfront collections.

- They minimize disputes and confusion regarding insurance coverage, reducing the need for retroactive adjustments or re-billing.

- They promote transparency in the financial aspect of healthcare services, improving patient satisfaction and trust.

Question 2: What information is typically verified during the insurance verification and eligibility checking process?

Answer: The information typically verified during the insurance verification and eligibility checking process includes:

- Validity of the insurance policy

- Policyholder details (if different from the patient)

- Coverage dates and effective dates of the policy

- In-network or out-of-network status of the provider

- Covered services, exclusions, and limitations

- Verification of pre-authorization or referral requirements (if applicable)

- Co-payment, deductible, and coinsurance amounts

- Coordination of benefits (if the patient has multiple insurance plans)

3. Patient Financial Responsibility and Estimation

Question 1: Why is patient financial responsibility estimation important in the revenue cycle management (RCM) process?

Answer: Patient financial responsibility estimation is important in the RCM process because:

- It helps patients understand their financial obligations for healthcare services in advance, improving transparency and reducing surprises.

- It enables proactive financial planning for both patients and healthcare organizations.

- It facilitates discussions about payment options, financial assistance programs, and available resources.

- It improves the likelihood of timely and accurate payment from patients, reducing bad debt and accounts receivable.

Question 2: What factors should be considered when estimating patient financial responsibility?

Answer: When estimating patient financial responsibility, the following factors should be considered:

- Insurance coverage details, including copayments, deductibles, and coinsurance.

- In-network or out-of-network status of the provider and its impact on patient cost-sharing.

- Coverage limitations, exclusions, or restrictions that may affect payment responsibilities.

- Any pre-authorization or referral requirements and associated costs.

- Coverage limits or maximums for specific services or treatment.

- Patient-specific factors such as the utilization of benefits, previous payments made, and outstanding balances.

These exercises provide an opportunity to reinforce the knowledge gained from the chapter on Patient Registration and Pre-Service Revenue Cycle. The questions assess understanding and reinforce key concepts related to patient pre-registration and demographic data collection, insurance verification and eligibility checking, and patient financial responsibility estimation in the revenue cycle management process.

5. Scheduling and Patient Access Management

5.1 Efficient Appointment Scheduling Strategies:

Efficient appointment scheduling is a crucial component of revenue cycle management and patient access management. Effective scheduling strategies help maximize provider productivity, optimize resource utilization, minimize wait times, and enhance patient satisfaction. Here are key considerations for implementing efficient appointment scheduling strategies:

1. Standardize Scheduling Processes:

Establish standardized scheduling processes and protocols across the organization. Define clear guidelines for scheduling appointments, including time slots, duration of appointments, and the allocation of specific appointment types. This promotes consistency and streamlines the scheduling workflow.

2. Use Advanced Scheduling Systems:

Utilize advanced scheduling systems or electronic health record (EHR) platforms with integrated scheduling functionalities. These systems can automate appointment scheduling, provide real-time availability, and facilitate easy rescheduling or cancellations. Leverage scheduling software that allows staff to view multiple providers' schedules simultaneously for efficient coordination.

3. Patient-Centric Scheduling:

Prioritize patient-centric scheduling by offering convenient and flexible appointment options. Consider extended hours, same-day appointments, telehealth options, and online self-scheduling capabilities. Accommodate patient preferences and work towards reducing wait times and improving access to care.

4. Prioritize Urgent and Preventive Appointments:

Ensure that urgent appointments and preventive care visits are given priority in the scheduling process. Allocate specific slots for urgent cases and preventive services to ensure timely access to care and address high-priority healthcare needs.

5. Streamline Appointment Types and Durations:

Optimize provider schedules by streamlining appointment types and durations. Analyze historical data to determine the average time required for different appointment types and adjust scheduling accordingly. This helps minimize overbooking or underutilization of provider time, enhancing productivity.

6. Implement Advanced Booking and Reminders:

Offer advanced booking options for routine appointments or follow-up visits. This enables patients to secure appointments well in advance, reducing last-minute scheduling challenges. Implement automated appointment reminders via phone, email, or text messages to minimize no-shows and late cancellations.

7. Manage Overbooking and Cancellations:

Develop policies and strategies to handle overbooking and cancellations effectively. Define protocols for managing appointment waitlists and rescheduling canceled appointments to optimize provider schedules and reduce gaps in the appointment calendar.

8. Consider Patient Complexity and Appointment Types:

Consider the complexity of patient needs and the required resources when scheduling appointments. Allocate appropriate time slots for patients requiring longer consultations, procedures, or specialized services. Balance provider workload and ensure adequate time for each patient encounter.

9. Monitor and Adjust Scheduling Performance:

Regularly monitor scheduling performance metrics, such as appointment adherence, patient wait times, and provider utilization rates. Analyze data to identify bottlenecks, inefficiencies, or areas for improvement. Make necessary adjustments to optimize scheduling practices and enhance patient access.

10. Communication and Patient Education:

Clearly communicate appointment expectations, including arrival times, necessary preparations, and any specific instructions or documentation required. Educate patients on the importance of adhering to scheduled appointments and the impact of no-shows on access to care.

11. Staff Training and Coordination:

Provide comprehensive training to staff members involved in appointment scheduling. Ensure they understand the scheduling protocols, system functionalities, and patient communication best practices. Foster effective coordination and communication among staff to address scheduling challenges and minimize errors.

Efficient appointment scheduling strategies not only optimize provider productivity and resource utilization but also enhance patient access and satisfaction. By implementing standardized processes, leveraging advanced scheduling systems, and prioritizing patient needs, healthcare organizations can streamline the scheduling process and improve revenue cycle management.

5.2 Patient Access Management Best Practices:

Patient access management encompasses various processes and practices that facilitate patient entry into the healthcare system, from scheduling appointments to registration and insurance verification. Implementing best practices in patient access management ensures a seamless patient experience, enhances revenue cycle efficiency, and improves overall operational performance. Here are key patient access management best practices:

1. Patient-Centered Approach:

Prioritize patient-centered care by placing patients' needs and preferences at the forefront. Foster a culture of empathy, respect, and responsiveness in all patient interactions. Ensure that the patient access team is trained to deliver excellent customer service and address patient concerns effectively.

2. Streamlined Patient Intake:

Streamline the patient intake process to minimize wait times and reduce administrative burden. Utilize technology solutions, such as online pre-registration and electronic forms, to collect patient information in advance. Automate data entry processes to eliminate manual errors and improve efficiency.

3. Centralized Scheduling and Registration:

Establish a centralized scheduling and registration system to ensure consistency and coordination across different service areas. Use integrated electronic systems that allow seamless transfer of patient information between departments, eliminating the need for redundant data entry.

4. Clear and Transparent Communication:

Communicate clearly and transparently with patients about appointment scheduling, insurance coverage, financial responsibilities, and any necessary preparations. Provide information in a language and format that patients can easily understand. Address any questions or concerns promptly to ensure patient satisfaction and engagement.

5. Proactive Insurance Verification:

Verify insurance coverage and eligibility before the patient's visit to minimize claim denials and patient billing issues. Implement real-time eligibility verification systems that allow instant access to insurance information. Regularly update and maintain accurate insurance data for each patient.

6. Financial Counseling and Assistance:

Offer financial counseling services to patients to help them navigate insurance coverage, understand their financial responsibilities, and explore available financial assistance programs. Provide guidance on payment options, eligibility for charity care or sliding fee scales, and available resources for financial support.

7. Staff Training and Education:

Invest in comprehensive training and education programs for the patient access team. Ensure staff members are well-versed in insurance policies, billing processes, patient communication, and legal requirements, such as HIPAA and compliance regulations. Ongoing training keeps staff updated on industry changes and best practices.

8. Performance Monitoring and Metrics:

Establish key performance indicators (KPIs) to measure patient access management performance. Monitor metrics such as appointment wait times, patient satisfaction scores, appointment utilization rates, and revenue cycle metrics. Regularly analyze data and identify areas for improvement.

9. Continuous Process Improvement:

Foster a culture of continuous process improvement in patient access management. Encourage staff to identify bottlenecks, inefficiencies, and opportunities for optimization. Implement feedback mechanisms and engage the patient access team in problem-solving and quality improvement initiatives.

10. Collaborative Interdepartmental Communication:

Promote collaboration and effective communication between patient access, clinical departments, billing, and other stakeholders. Facilitate regular meetings and share relevant information to enhance coordination, address challenges, and align goals across departments.

11. Technology Adoption:

Leverage technology solutions, such as electronic health record (EHR) systems, patient portals, and self-service kiosks, to streamline patient access processes. Implement automated appointment reminders, online scheduling, and virtual check-in options to improve efficiency and patient convenience.

Implementing these best practices in patient access management enhances the patient experience, streamlines revenue cycle operations, and improves overall organizational performance. By focusing on patient-centered care, effective communication, streamlined processes, and continuous improvement, healthcare organizations can optimize patient access and drive positive outcomes.

5.3 Reducing No-Shows and Cancellations:

No-shows and cancellations can disrupt the patient schedule, result in lost revenue, and lead to inefficiencies in the healthcare system. Implementing strategies to reduce no-shows and cancellations improves patient access, optimizes resource utilization, and enhances the overall revenue cycle management. Here are key considerations for reducing no-shows and cancellations:

1. Clear Appointment Reminders:

Implement a robust appointment reminder system that utilizes multiple communication channels, such as phone calls, text messages, and emails, to remind patients of their upcoming appointments. Reminders should include the appointment date, time, location, and any necessary instructions or preparations.

2. Advance Reminders:

Send appointment reminders well in advance to allow patients sufficient time to reschedule or prepare for their appointments. Sending reminders 24 to 48 hours in advance helps reduce the likelihood of patients forgetting or missing their scheduled visits.

3. Confirmations and Follow-ups:

Implement a confirmation process that requires patients to confirm their attendance a day or two before their scheduled appointments. Follow up with patients who have not confirmed to determine their intent to attend or reschedule the appointment.

4. Telephonic Confirmation Calls:

Consider making telephonic confirmation calls to patients who have not confirmed their appointments. This personal touch can help re-engage patients, address any concerns or barriers they may have, and provide an opportunity to reschedule if needed.

5. Waitlist Management:

Implement a waitlist management system to fill vacant appointment slots due to cancellations or rescheduling. When patients cancel or reschedule, proactively contact patients on the waitlist to offer them the newly available appointment times.

6. Overbooking Management:

Develop a strategy for managing overbooking to minimize appointment gaps. Implement a system that carefully tracks patient preferences, appointment durations, and provider availability to optimize the scheduling process. Overbooking should be done judiciously to avoid overwhelming providers and compromising patient care.

7. Patient Education:

Educate patients on the importance of honoring their appointments and the impact of no-shows and cancellations on access to care and overall healthcare operations. Emphasize the value of their time, as well as the time and resources of the healthcare providers and staff.

8. Reminder Customization:

Customize appointment reminders based on patient preferences and communication preferences. Offer options for patients to receive reminders via their preferred channels, such as text messages, emails, or phone calls. Allow patients to opt-in to their preferred method of communication.

9. Financial Consequences:

Clearly communicate the financial consequences of no-shows and late cancellations to patients. Inform them about any applicable fees or penalties for missed appointments or short notice cancellations. Ensure that the financial policies are communicated and understood during the appointment scheduling process.

10. Patient Engagement Strategies:

Implement patient engagement strategies to foster patient commitment to their appointments. Engage patients in their healthcare journey through education, reminders of the importance of continuity of care, and personalized communication that highlights the benefits of attending appointments.

11. Data Analysis and Quality Improvement:

Regularly analyze data on no-shows and cancellations to identify patterns, trends, and common reasons for missed appointments. Use this information to drive quality improvement initiatives and implement targeted interventions, such as patient education campaigns or scheduling process modifications.

By implementing these strategies, healthcare organizations can effectively reduce no-shows and cancellations, optimize appointment utilization, and enhance revenue cycle management. Consistent communication, proactive patient engagement, and continuous process improvement contribute to improved patient access and overall operational efficiency.

1. Efficient Appointment Scheduling Strategies

Question 1: Why is efficient appointment scheduling important in the revenue cycle management (RCM) process?

Answer: Efficient appointment scheduling is important in the RCM process because:

- It maximizes the utilization of healthcare providers' time and resources, improving operational efficiency.

- It reduces patient wait times and improves overall patient satisfaction.

- It helps minimize gaps and optimize the schedule to ensure a steady flow of patients, reducing idle time and maximizing revenue potential.

- It allows for appropriate allocation of resources, such as specialized equipment or staff, based on the scheduled appointments.

- It facilitates accurate forecasting of patient volume and workload, enabling efficient staff allocation and capacity planning.

Question 2: What are some efficient appointment scheduling strategies that healthcare organizations can employ?

Answer: Healthcare organizations can employ the following efficient appointment scheduling strategies:

- Implementing advanced scheduling systems and tools that allow for automated scheduling, real-time availability, and patient self-scheduling options.

- Implementing scheduling protocols that prioritize urgent or high-priority appointments, ensuring timely access for patients in need.

- Optimizing provider schedules to balance patient demand, provider availability, and appointment durations, reducing gaps and maximizing productivity.

- Offering convenient scheduling options, such as online scheduling, phone appointments, or extended hours, to accommodate patient preferences and increase access.

- Implementing reminder systems, such as automated appointment reminders via phone, text, or email, to reduce no-shows and improve patient attendance rates.

- Conducting regular reviews and analysis of scheduling data to identify bottlenecks, trends, and areas for improvement.

2. Patient Access Management Best Practices

Question 1: Why is effective patient access management important in the revenue cycle management (RCM) process?

Answer: Effective patient access management is important in the RCM process because:

- It ensures that patients have timely access to healthcare services, reducing delays in care and improving patient outcomes.

- It facilitates accurate patient registration, insurance verification, and eligibility checking, setting the foundation for a smooth revenue cycle process.

- It helps prevent financial barriers and improves upfront collections by proactively identifying patient financial responsibilities and discussing payment options.

- It reduces administrative errors and avoids billing issues by capturing accurate and complete patient information at the point of access.

- It enhances patient satisfaction by providing a positive and efficient experience from the initial point of contact with the healthcare organization.

Question 2: What are some patient access management best practices that healthcare organizations can implement?

Answer: Healthcare organizations can implement the following patient access management best practices:

- Streamlining registration processes to minimize paperwork and improve efficiency, such as utilizing electronic forms or self-check-in kiosks.

- Training staff on effective communication and customer service skills to create a welcoming and supportive environment for patients.

- Implementing technology solutions, such as electronic health records (EHRs) and patient portals, to facilitate access to patient information and streamline documentation processes.

- Ensuring staff are well-trained on insurance verification and eligibility checking procedures, including knowledge of different insurance plans and coverage requirements.

- Implementing proactive financial counseling and patient education programs to inform patients about their financial responsibilities, available resources, and payment options.

- Utilizing data analytics to identify scheduling patterns, optimize patient flow, and allocate resources effectively.

- Implementing efficient referral management processes to ensure timely access to specialists and coordinated care.

3. Reducing No-Shows and Cancellations

Question 1: Why is reducing no-shows and cancellations important in the revenue cycle management (RCM) process?

Answer: Reducing no-shows and cancellations is important in the RCM process because:

- It minimizes lost revenue from missed appointments and unutilized provider time slots.

- It improves resource utilization by ensuring that appointment slots are allocated to patients who will attend, maximizing productivity.

- It allows for better patient access by reducing wait times and enabling other patients to receive timely care.

- It improves patient satisfaction by reducing the need for rescheduling and inconvenience caused by no-shows or last-minute cancellations.

- It facilitates accurate scheduling, improves workflow efficiency, and minimizes disruptions in the revenue cycle process.

Question 2: What are some strategies that healthcare organizations can employ to reduce no-shows and cancellations?

Answer: Healthcare organizations can employ the following strategies to reduce no-shows and cancellations:

- Implementing appointment reminder systems, such as automated phone calls, text messages, or email reminders, to provide patients with timely reminders of their upcoming appointments.

- Offering multiple communication channels for appointment reminders, allowing patients to choose their preferred method of receiving reminders.

- Implementing policies and procedures that clearly communicate the organization's expectations regarding appointment attendance and cancellation.

- Offering flexible rescheduling options to accommodate patients who need to change their appointments, reducing the likelihood of cancellations.

- Implementing overbooking or waitlist management strategies to fill appointment slots in case of last-minute cancellations or no-shows.

- Analyzing data and monitoring appointment patterns to identify trends and factors contributing to no-shows and cancellations, enabling targeted interventions and improvement efforts.

- Providing patient education on the importance of attending scheduled appointments and the impact of no-shows on healthcare delivery and access.

These exercises provide an opportunity to reinforce the knowledge gained from the chapter on Scheduling and Patient Access Management. The questions assess understanding and reinforce key concepts related to efficient appointment scheduling strategies, patient access management best practices, and strategies for reducing no-shows and cancellations in the revenue cycle management process.

6. Medical Coding and Documentation

6.1 Introduction to Medical Coding Systems (CPT, ICD, HCPCS):

Medical coding is a vital aspect of revenue cycle management, ensuring accurate documentation and billing for healthcare services. Understanding the different coding systems is essential for coding professionals, healthcare providers, and billing staff. Let's explore the three primary coding systems used in healthcare: Current Procedural Terminology (CPT), International Classification of Diseases (ICD), and Healthcare Common Procedure Coding System (HCPCS).

1. Current Procedural Terminology (CPT):

CPT is a coding system developed and maintained by the American Medical Association (AMA). It is primarily used to describe medical procedures and services provided by healthcare professionals in the United States. CPT codes are numeric and consist of five digits. Each code represents a specific medical procedure, service, or test.

CPT codes are categorized into three main sections:

a. Evaluation and Management (E&M): E&M codes are used to report patient encounters, such as office visits, consultations, and hospital visits. These codes capture the complexity and level of the patient encounter, considering factors like history taking, examination, medical decision-making, and time spent.

b. Surgical Procedures: Surgical procedure codes describe surgical interventions, including both minor and major surgeries. Each surgical code specifies the procedure, anatomical location, approach, and any associated services or modifiers.

c. Ancillary Services: Ancillary service codes encompass a range of services, such as laboratory tests, diagnostic imaging, vaccinations, physical therapy, and other non-surgical procedures. These codes capture the specific service provided and may include additional modifiers or add-on codes.

2. International Classification of Diseases (ICD):

The International Classification of Diseases (ICD) is a standardized system developed by the World Health Organization (WHO) for documenting and classifying diseases, conditions, and injuries. The current version used worldwide is ICD-10. ICD codes are alphanumeric and consist of up to seven characters.

ICD codes are used to capture diagnoses and reasons for patient encounters. They provide a common language for describing diseases and conditions, facilitating data collection, research, and analysis. ICD codes are essential for accurate reimbursement, statistical reporting, and population health monitoring.

ICD-10 codes are organized into chapters based on body systems and include codes for specific diseases, conditions, signs, symptoms, and external causes of injury or illness.

3. Healthcare Common Procedure Coding System (HCPCS):

HCPCS is a coding system used in the United States to report healthcare services, supplies, and equipment not covered by CPT codes. It is divided into two levels: Level I and Level II.

a. Level I HCPCS: Level I HCPCS codes are identical to CPT codes and are used to report physician services, procedures, and supplies. These codes are maintained and updated by the American Medical Association (AMA).

b. Level II HCPCS: Level II HCPCS codes are alphanumeric and are used to report non-physician services, durable medical equipment (DME), supplies, drugs, and other healthcare services not covered by Level I codes. These codes are maintained by the Centers for Medicare and Medicaid Services (CMS).

Level II HCPCS codes are further divided into sections, including durable medical equipment, drugs, supplies, ambulance services, and more.

Accurate and detailed coding using CPT, ICD, and HCPCS codes is crucial for proper reimbursement, claims processing, and compliance with healthcare regulations. It requires a solid understanding of these coding systems, continuous education, and adherence to coding guidelines and documentation requirements.

6.2 Accurate Documentation and Coding Guidelines:

Accurate documentation is essential for proper medical coding and billing, as it ensures that the services provided are appropriately captured and billed for reimbursement. Adhering to coding guidelines and best practices improves coding accuracy, reduces claim denials, and supports compliant billing practices. Here are key considerations for accurate documentation and coding:

1. Thorough and Complete Documentation:

Healthcare providers should strive for thorough and complete documentation of patient encounters, including relevant medical history, examination findings, diagnoses, and treatments provided. Clear and detailed documentation supports accurate code assignment and reflects the complexity and severity of the patient's condition.

2. Specificity and Detail:

Document diagnoses and procedures with specificity and detail. Avoid using vague or unspecified terms when more specific terms are available. Provide sufficient information to accurately describe the patient's condition or procedure, supporting the appropriate code assignment.

3. Use of Standard Terminology:

Utilize standard medical terminology and coding conventions to describe diagnoses, procedures, and other clinical information. Familiarize yourself with coding guidelines and coding resources to ensure consistency and accuracy in the documentation and coding process.

4. Linkage between Diagnosis and Procedure:

Establish a clear linkage between the documented diagnosis and the procedures performed or services provided. Ensure that the documented diagnosis justifies the necessity and medical appropriateness of the procedures, tests, or treatments billed.

5. Compliance with Official Guidelines:

Adhere to the official coding guidelines published by the coding authorities, such as the American Medical Association (AMA), the Centers for Medicare and Medicaid Services (CMS), and the World Health Organization (WHO) for CPT, ICD, and HCPCS coding. Stay updated with any revisions or changes to coding guidelines.

6. Consistent and Timely Documentation:

Ensure that documentation is consistent, timely, and completed promptly after patient encounters. Delayed or incomplete documentation can lead to inaccuracies in code assignment and billing, potentially impacting reimbursement and compliance.

7. Documenting Medical Necessity:

Clearly document the medical necessity of procedures and services provided. Include information that supports the medical reason for the intervention, demonstrating that it is appropriate and required for the patient's diagnosis or condition.

8. Accurate Time-Based Documentation:

For services billed based on time, such as time-based E&M codes, document the actual time spent with the patient, including face-to-face time and non-face-to-face activities. Accurate time documentation ensures proper code selection and billing.

9. Ongoing Education and Training:

Continuously educate and train healthcare providers, coding professionals, and billing staff on coding guidelines, documentation requirements, and updates in coding practices. Stay informed about changes in coding regulations, reimbursement policies, and compliance standards.

10. Auditing and Compliance Review:

Regularly conduct internal audits and compliance reviews to assess coding accuracy, identify documentation gaps or errors, and ensure compliance with coding and billing regulations. Address any identified issues promptly and implement corrective actions.

11. Collaboration and Communication:

Foster effective communication and collaboration between healthcare providers, coding professionals, and billing staff. Encourage open dialogue to address documentation and coding-related concerns, clarify coding guidelines, and share best practices.

Accurate documentation and coding are critical for proper reimbursement, compliance, and quality healthcare delivery. By following coding guidelines, maintaining thorough documentation, and promoting ongoing education, healthcare organizations can improve coding accuracy, reduce claim denials, and optimize revenue cycle management.

6.3 Risk Adjustment Coding in RCM:

Risk adjustment coding plays a significant role in revenue cycle management, particularly in healthcare systems that utilize risk adjustment models for reimbursement. Risk adjustment coding is used to account for the health status and predicted costs of treating patients, ensuring fair and accurate payment for healthcare services. Here are key considerations for risk adjustment coding in RCM:

1. Understanding Risk Adjustment:

Risk adjustment is a method used to modify reimbursement rates based on the predicted healthcare costs associated with individual patients. It takes into account factors such as age, gender, health conditions, and comorbidities to adjust payments appropriately. Risk adjustment ensures that healthcare providers are adequately compensated for treating patients with higher healthcare needs and costs.

2. Hierarchical Condition Category (HCC) Coding:

Hierarchical Condition Category (HCC) coding is a common risk adjustment model used by many healthcare systems. HCC coding involves assigning codes to specific diagnoses or health conditions based on their severity and expected impact on healthcare costs. The HCC codes are hierarchical, meaning that more severe or chronic conditions have higher-weighted codes, leading to higher reimbursement.

3. Accurate Diagnosis Coding:

Accurate diagnosis coding is crucial for risk adjustment. It is important to document and code all relevant diagnoses and health conditions that are present and impact the patient's healthcare needs. Ensure that the coding captures the specificity and severity of the conditions to reflect the appropriate HCC codes.

4. Complete Documentation:

Complete documentation of the patient's health conditions, comorbidities, and complications is essential for risk adjustment coding. Providers should thoroughly document the patient's medical history, current conditions, and any significant changes or developments to support accurate code assignment.

5. Coding Documentation Guidelines:

Follow coding documentation guidelines specific to risk adjustment coding. These guidelines may differ from standard coding guidelines and may include additional requirements for capturing specific details, severity levels, or timeframes related to health conditions.

6. Ongoing Review and Updating of Codes:

Regularly review and update risk adjustment codes as the patient's health status changes over time. Continuously monitor the patient's conditions, treatments, and outcomes to ensure accurate and up-to-date coding. This helps reflect the patient's evolving healthcare needs and supports appropriate reimbursement.

7. Collaboration between Providers and Coders:

Foster collaboration and communication between healthcare providers and coders to ensure accurate risk adjustment coding. Providers should document and communicate relevant clinical information, while coders should seek clarification and additional details when necessary to ensure coding accuracy.

8. Compliance with Coding and Billing Regulations:

Ensure compliance with coding and billing regulations related to risk adjustment coding. Stay updated with changes in coding guidelines, reimbursement policies, and compliance standards specific to risk adjustment. Implement internal auditing and monitoring processes to identify and address any coding or documentation deficiencies.

9. Training and Education:

Provide training and education to coding professionals and healthcare providers on risk adjustment coding. Keep them informed about the latest coding guidelines, documentation requirements, and updates in risk adjustment methodologies. Ongoing education helps ensure coding accuracy and compliance.

10. Utilize Technology Solutions:

Leverage technology solutions, such as coding software and electronic health record (EHR) systems, that support risk adjustment coding. These tools can assist in identifying and assigning appropriate codes based on the patient's clinical information, enhancing coding accuracy and efficiency.

Risk adjustment coding is essential for fair and accurate reimbursement in healthcare systems that utilize risk adjustment models. By adhering to coding and documentation guidelines, collaborating effectively, and staying updated with coding regulations, healthcare organizations can optimize risk adjustment coding in revenue cycle management.

Exercise 6: Medical Coding and Documentation

1. Introduction to Medical Coding Systems (CPT, ICD, HCPCS)

Question 1: What are the primary purposes of medical coding systems, such as CPT, ICD, and HCPCS?

Answer: The primary purposes of medical coding systems are:

- CPT (Current Procedural Terminology): CPT codes are used to describe medical procedures and services performed by healthcare providers. They allow for standardized documentation and billing of services rendered, ensuring accurate reimbursement and facilitating data analysis.

- ICD (International Classification of Diseases): ICD codes are used to classify and code diagnoses, symptoms, and inpatient procedures. They provide a standardized way of documenting and reporting medical conditions, enabling accurate billing, epidemiological studies, and healthcare data analysis.

- HCPCS (Healthcare Common Procedure Coding System): HCPCS codes are used primarily for coding procedures, services, and supplies not covered by CPT codes. They include durable medical equipment, prosthetics, orthotics, and supplies. HCPCS codes are used for billing purposes, ensuring appropriate reimbursement.

Question 2: Describe the difference between CPT, ICD, and HCPCS codes.

Answer: The difference between CPT, ICD, and HCPCS codes lies in their purpose and the types of information they capture:

- CPT codes: CPT codes capture the procedures and services provided by healthcare professionals, such as surgeries, office visits, and diagnostic tests. They provide a standardized way to document and bill for these services.

- ICD codes: ICD codes capture diagnoses, symptoms, and inpatient procedures. They classify and code medical conditions based on a standardized system, facilitating data analysis, epidemiological studies, and accurate billing for patient encounters.

- HCPCS codes: HCPCS codes are used for procedures, services, and supplies not covered by CPT codes. They primarily apply to durable medical equipment, prosthetics, orthotics, and supplies. HCPCS codes ensure accurate billing and reimbursement for these items.

2. Accurate Documentation and Coding Guidelines

Question 1: Why is accurate documentation essential for proper medical coding and billing?

Answer: Accurate documentation is essential for proper medical coding and billing because:

- It ensures that the services provided are accurately captured and coded, leading to appropriate reimbursement.

- It supports medical necessity by providing a clear and comprehensive record of the patient's condition and the services rendered.

- It facilitates accurate claims submission, reducing the risk of denials or delays in reimbursement.

- It ensures compliance with coding guidelines and regulations set by payers and regulatory bodies.

- It supports continuity of care by providing a detailed record of the patient's medical history and treatment.

Question 2: What are some important guidelines for accurate documentation and coding in healthcare?

Answer: Important guidelines for accurate documentation and coding in healthcare include:

- Use clear, concise, and specific language to describe the patient's condition, services provided, and outcomes.

- Document all relevant details, including the patient's signs, symptoms, medical history, and any associated comorbidities.

- Use appropriate terminology and coding conventions as specified by the coding systems (CPT, ICD, HCPCS).

- Ensure that the documentation supports the medical necessity of the services provided.

- Include the date, time, and provider signature or electronic attestation for all entries.

- Avoid using abbreviations or acronyms that may be misunderstood or lead to coding errors.

- Regularly update and revise documentation to reflect changes in the patient's condition or treatment plan.

3. Risk Adjustment Coding in RCM

Question 1: What is risk adjustment coding, and why is it important in revenue cycle management (RCM)?

Answer: Risk adjustment coding is a method used in healthcare to account for the differences in patient complexity and health status when determining reimbursement. It involves assigning diagnostic codes that reflect the severity of illness or chronic conditions. Risk adjustment coding is important in RCM because:

- It ensures that reimbursement accurately reflects the patient's level of risk and the resources required to provide care.

- It supports fair and equitable reimbursement by accounting for differences in patient population characteristics.

- It promotes accurate reporting and analysis of healthcare data, enabling better assessment of outcomes and quality of care.

- It helps manage financial risk by accurately predicting and adjusting for the cost of caring for patients with high-risk conditions.

Question 2: What are some examples of risk adjustment models used in healthcare?

Answer: Some examples of risk adjustment models used in healthcare include:

- Hierarchical Condition Category (HCC): HCC is used by Medicare Advantage and other healthcare payers to adjust reimbursement based on the patient's demographic information, diagnoses, and conditions.

- Clinical Risk Groups (CRG): CRG is a risk adjustment model that categorizes patients based on their age, gender, diagnoses, and healthcare resource utilization.

- Chronic Illness and Disability Payment System (CDPS): CDPS is used by Medicaid programs to adjust payments for individuals with disabilities or chronic conditions based on their diagnosis and functional status.

These exercises provide an opportunity to reinforce the knowledge gained from the chapter on Medical Coding and Documentation. The questions assess understanding and reinforce key concepts related to the introduction to medical coding systems (CPT, ICD, HCPCS), accurate documentation and coding guidelines, and risk adjustment coding in revenue cycle management.

7. Charge Capture and Reimbursement

7.1 Importance of Charge Capture in RCM:

Charge capture is a critical component of revenue cycle management (RCM) that ensures accurate recording and capturing of services provided to patients. It involves the timely and accurate documentation of all billable services, procedures, and supplies delivered by healthcare providers. Effective charge capture processes are essential for maximizing reimbursement, reducing revenue leakage, and maintaining financial stability. Here are key considerations for understanding the importance of charge capture in RCM:

1. Revenue Maximization:

Accurate and timely charge capture is crucial for maximizing revenue in healthcare organizations. By capturing all billable services and supplies, providers can ensure that they are appropriately reimbursed for the care provided. Failure to capture charges or undercoding can result in revenue loss and financial strain on the organization.

2. Compliance and Audit Readiness:

Proper charge capture practices help ensure compliance with coding and billing regulations, reducing the risk of fraudulent or erroneous billing. By accurately documenting and capturing charges, healthcare organizations can be prepared for audits and demonstrate the appropriate utilization of resources and services.

3. Documentation Integrity:

Charge capture requires accurate documentation of services provided, including procedures performed, supplies used, and any relevant clinical details. This promotes documentation integrity, supporting the accuracy and completeness of the patient's medical record.

4. Efficient Claims Processing:

Effective charge capture processes streamline claims processing and reduce claim denials. Timely and accurate charge capture ensures that claims are complete and contain the necessary information for reimbursement. This minimizes delays in payment and reduces the administrative burden of claim resubmissions.

5. Revenue Cycle Efficiency:

Charge capture is a fundamental step in the revenue cycle, ensuring that services provided are appropriately coded, billed, and reimbursed. Efficient charge capture processes improve revenue cycle efficiency by reducing manual errors, streamlining workflows, and optimizing cash flow.

6. Improved Billing Accuracy:

Accurate charge capture contributes to improved billing accuracy, reducing the risk of billing errors and claim rejections. By capturing charges correctly the first time, healthcare organizations can enhance billing accuracy, leading to faster and more accurate reimbursement.

7. Enhanced Financial Performance:

Proper charge capture practices support overall financial performance by minimizing revenue leakage and optimizing reimbursement. When charges are accurately captured and billed, healthcare organizations can maintain financial stability, invest in resources, and deliver quality patient care.

8. Collaboration and Communication:

Effective charge capture requires collaboration and communication among healthcare providers, coding professionals, and billing staff. Clear and timely communication ensures that all billable services and supplies are appropriately documented and captured. Collaboration helps identify and resolve any coding or documentation issues that may impact revenue.

9. Technology Integration:

Leveraging technology solutions, such as electronic health record (EHR) systems and charge capture software, streamlines the charge capture process. These tools automate charge capture, improve coding accuracy, and facilitate real-time documentation, ensuring charges are captured promptly and accurately.

10. Continuous Process Improvement:

Regularly review and evaluate charge capture processes to identify areas for improvement. Monitor key performance indicators (KPIs) such as charge lag, charge capture rate, and denial rates to assess the effectiveness of charge capture practices. Implement process improvements to enhance revenue cycle performance.

Accurate and efficient charge capture is vital for revenue optimization, compliance, and financial stability in healthcare organizations. By prioritizing charge capture processes, implementing technology solutions, and fostering collaboration, healthcare organizations can maximize reimbursement and ensure a robust revenue cycle management system.

Proper documentation and coding are essential for accurate charge capture in revenue cycle management. Accurate and detailed documentation of the services provided ensures that the appropriate codes are assigned, leading to accurate billing and reimbursement. Here are key considerations for documentation and coding to facilitate proper charge capture:

1. Complete and Detailed Documentation:

Healthcare providers should ensure complete and detailed documentation of all services rendered. Document the patient's medical history, chief complaint, physical examination findings, diagnostic tests, procedures performed, and any additional relevant information. Comprehensive documentation supports accurate code assignment and appropriate charge capture.

2. Specificity in Diagnosis Coding:

Assign the most specific diagnosis codes that describe the patient's condition or reason for the encounter. Utilize the appropriate level of specificity available in the coding system (e.g., ICD-10) to capture the exact nature of the diagnosis. Specific diagnosis coding is crucial for accurate charge capture and appropriate reimbursement.

3. Accurate Procedure Coding:

Code procedures accurately based on the documentation of the services provided. Utilize the appropriate coding system (e.g., CPT or HCPCS) to assign codes for each procedure performed. Document the details of the procedure, including the approach, technique, and any additional modifiers or applicable codes.

4. Linkage between Documentation and Codes:

Establish a clear linkage between the documented services and the assigned codes. Ensure that the codes selected accurately represent the documented procedures, treatments, and supplies provided to the patient. The documentation should support the medical necessity and appropriateness of the assigned codes.

5. Compliance with Coding Guidelines:

Adhere to coding guidelines and conventions outlined by coding authorities, such as the American Medical Association (AMA) and the Centers for Medicare and Medicaid Services (CMS). Stay updated with any revisions or updates to the coding guidelines to ensure compliance and accurate code assignment.

6. Documentation of Unbilled Services:

Avoid missing or omitting documentation of services provided, as this can lead to revenue loss. Implement processes to capture and document all billable services promptly. Regularly review encounter documentation to ensure that all services are captured for appropriate coding and billing.

7. Ongoing Education and Training:

Provide education and training to healthcare providers, coding professionals, and billing staff on proper documentation practices and coding guidelines. Continuous education helps maintain coding accuracy, promotes consistent documentation standards, and enhances charge capture processes.

8. Collaboration and Communication:

Foster collaboration and effective communication between healthcare providers, coding professionals, and billing staff. Encourage open dialogue to address documentation and coding-related queries, clarify coding guidelines, and resolve any discrepancies. Timely and accurate communication ensures proper charge capture.

9. Technology Integration:

Leverage technology solutions, such as electronic health record (EHR) systems and coding software, to facilitate accurate documentation and coding. These tools streamline the coding process, provide coding guidance, and improve accuracy and efficiency in charge capture.

10. Regular Auditing and Quality Assurance:

Conduct regular internal audits and quality assurance checks to ensure the accuracy and completeness of documentation and coding. Perform coding audits to identify any coding errors or discrepancies and implement corrective measures as necessary. This helps optimize charge capture accuracy and compliance.

By prioritizing complete and accurate documentation, following coding guidelines, promoting collaboration, and leveraging technology, healthcare organizations can facilitate proper charge capture in revenue cycle management. Proper charge capture ensures accurate billing, appropriate reimbursement, and optimized revenue cycle performance.

Reimbursement methodologies and rates determine how healthcare providers are paid for the services they render. Understanding different reimbursement methodologies and rates is crucial for revenue cycle management. Here are key considerations regarding reimbursement methodologies and rates:

1. Fee-for-Service (FFS):

Fee-for-service is a traditional reimbursement model where healthcare providers are paid based on the individual services provided to patients. Each service or procedure is assigned a specific fee, typically based on a fee schedule. Providers submit claims for each service rendered, and payment is made based on the fee schedule or negotiated rates with payers.

Under the fee-for-service model, providers are reimbursed for each service based on the agreed-upon rate, which may vary depending on factors such as geographical location, payer contracts, and the provider's specialty.

2. Diagnosis-Related Groups (DRGs):

Diagnosis-Related Groups is a reimbursement methodology commonly used for inpatient hospital services. Patients with similar diagnoses, treatments, and resources utilized are grouped into specific categories known as DRGs. Providers receive a fixed reimbursement amount for each DRG, regardless of the actual costs incurred during the patient's stay. DRGs are based on a predetermined rate that considers factors such as diagnosis, procedures, patient demographics, and severity of illness.

DRG reimbursement encourages efficiency and cost containment by incentivizing providers to deliver care within the fixed payment amount while maintaining quality standards.

3. Capitation:

Capitation is a reimbursement methodology in which providers receive a fixed, per-member, per-month (PMPM) payment from a payer or health plan. Providers are paid a predetermined amount for each enrolled patient, regardless of the actual services rendered or the frequency of patient visits. The capitation payment is intended to cover a defined set of services over a specified time period.

Capitation reimbursement places financial risk on providers, as they are responsible for delivering all necessary care within the allocated payment, irrespective of the actual costs incurred. It encourages preventive care, coordination, and efficient resource utilization.

4. Value-Based Reimbursement (VBR):

Value-based reimbursement is an evolving reimbursement methodology that focuses on the quality and outcomes of care rather than the quantity of services provided. Providers are rewarded based on predefined quality metrics, such as patient satisfaction, clinical outcomes, cost savings, and adherence to evidence-based guidelines.

Value-based reimbursement models include pay-for-performance (P4P), shared savings programs, bundled payments, and accountable care organizations (ACOs). These models incentivize providers to deliver high-quality, cost-effective care while improving patient outcomes.

5. Relative Value Units (RVUs):

Relative Value Units are a standard measurement used to determine the value or weight of specific medical services. RVUs consider the physician's work, practice expenses, and malpractice costs associated with a particular service. Each service is assigned a specific RVU value, which is then multiplied by a conversion factor to determine the reimbursement amount.

RVUs are commonly used in the fee-for-service model to establish reimbursement rates for various procedures and services. The Centers for Medicare and Medicaid Services (CMS) assigns RVUs to CPT codes for Medicare reimbursement, and private payers may also utilize RVUs as part of their reimbursement methodologies.

It is important for healthcare organizations to understand the reimbursement methodologies and rates utilized by different payers, including government programs (e.g., Medicare and Medicaid) and commercial insurance companies. This knowledge allows providers to optimize revenue cycle management, negotiate favorable contracts, and adapt their financial strategies accordingly. Additionally, staying updated with changes in reimbursement methodologies and rates helps providers navigate the evolving healthcare reimbursement landscape.

Exercise 7: Charge Capture and Reimbursement

1. Importance of Charge Capture in RCM

Question 1: Why is charge capture important in the revenue cycle management (RCM) process?

Answer: Charge capture is important in the RCM process because:

- It ensures accurate and complete capture of services provided by healthcare providers, allowing for proper billing and reimbursement.

- It facilitates proper documentation of services, which is crucial for compliance with coding and billing regulations.

- It maximizes revenue potential by capturing all billable services, preventing undercoding and missed revenue opportunities.

- It supports accurate claims submission, reducing the risk of denials or delays in reimbursement.

- It provides a basis for financial analysis and reporting, enabling organizations to assess the financial performance of specific services or departments.

Question 2: What are the potential consequences of inadequate or incomplete charge capture?

Answer: Inadequate or incomplete charge capture can have several potential consequences, including:

- Revenue loss: Missed or undercoded charges can result in lost revenue for healthcare organizations.

- Compliance issues: Incomplete or inaccurate charge capture can lead to non-compliance with coding and billing regulations, potentially resulting in legal and financial penalties.

- Claims denials: Inadequate charge capture may lead to denials or delays in reimbursement due to incomplete or incorrect documentation.

- Inaccurate financial reporting: Incomplete charge capture can impact financial reporting and analysis, leading to inaccurate assessments of revenue, costs, and profitability.

- Decreased patient satisfaction: Incomplete or inaccurate charge capture can result in incorrect billing or unexpected costs for patients, leading to dissatisfaction and potential reputational issues for the organization.

2. Documentation and Coding for Proper Charge Capture

Question 1: How does accurate documentation and coding contribute to proper charge capture in the revenue cycle management (RCM) process?

Answer: Accurate documentation and coding contribute to proper charge capture in the RCM process by:

- Ensuring that the services provided are accurately documented and coded, enabling accurate billing and reimbursement.

- Providing a clear and comprehensive record of the patient encounter, including the services performed, the complexity of the case, and any necessary supporting documentation.

- Facilitating compliance with coding and billing guidelines and regulations, reducing the risk of audit findings or denials.

- Enabling accurate claims submission by ensuring that the appropriate codes are assigned based on the documented services and diagnoses.

- Supporting medical necessity by documenting the reasons for performing the services and justifying the need for reimbursement.

- Promoting consistency and accuracy in charge capture by adhering to coding conventions, guidelines, and best practices.

Question 2: What are some important considerations for documentation and coding to support proper charge capture?

Answer: Some important considerations for documentation and coding to support proper charge capture include:

- Capturing all services performed during the patient encounter, including procedures, diagnostic tests, consultations, and treatments.

- Documenting the appropriate level of detail, specificity, and supporting documentation required for each service or procedure.

- Assigning the correct codes based on the documented services and diagnoses, using the appropriate code set (e.g., CPT, ICD, HCPCS).

- Ensuring that the documentation supports medical necessity and justifies the need for the services performed.

- Adhering to coding guidelines, conventions, and modifiers as specified by coding systems and payer requirements.

- Regularly updating and reviewing coding practices to stay current with changes in coding guidelines and regulations.

3. Reimbursement Methodologies and Rates

Question 1: What are the different reimbursement methodologies commonly used in healthcare?

Answer: Different reimbursement methodologies commonly used in healthcare include:

- Fee-for-Service (FFS): In FFS reimbursement, providers are paid a set fee for each service or procedure performed. The reimbursement amount is based on the provider's fee schedule or a negotiated rate with the payer.

- Diagnosis-Related Groups (DRGs): DRGs are a reimbursement methodology primarily used for inpatient hospital services. Payments are based on a predetermined rate assigned to specific diagnoses or conditions.

- Capitation: In capitation, providers receive a fixed payment per patient enrolled in a health plan, regardless of the services rendered. This methodology transfers financial risk from payers to providers.

- Bundled Payments: Bundled payments involve a single payment for multiple services provided during a defined episode of care. Providers are accountable for the quality and cost of care within that episode.

Question 2: What factors can influence reimbursement rates in healthcare?

Answer: Several factors can influence reimbursement rates in healthcare, including:

- Payer contracts and fee schedules: Reimbursement rates may be influenced by negotiated contracts and fee schedules between providers and payers.

- Government regulations and policies: Reimbursement rates for government programs such as Medicare and Medicaid are set by regulatory bodies and may be subject to legislative changes or updates.

- Healthcare market dynamics: Reimbursement rates can be influenced by supply and demand dynamics, regional variations in healthcare costs, and competition among providers.

- Quality and performance measures: Some reimbursement models include performance-based incentives or penalties tied to quality and outcome measures.

- Coding accuracy and documentation: Accurate coding and documentation impact the accuracy of reimbursement rates, as they form the basis for claims submission and payment calculation.

These exercises provide an opportunity to reinforce the knowledge gained from the chapter on Charge Capture and Reimbursement. The questions assess understanding and reinforce key concepts related to the importance of charge capture in RCM, documentation and coding for proper charge capture, and different reimbursement methodologies and rates in healthcare.

8. Claims Submission and Adjudication

8.1 Claims Submission Process and Requirements:

The claims submission process is a crucial step in revenue cycle management that involves submitting accurate and complete claims to payers for reimbursement. Understanding the claims submission process and meeting the requirements set by payers is essential for efficient revenue cycle operations. Here are key considerations for the claims submission process and its requirements:

1. Patient and Insurance Verification:

Before submitting a claim, verify the patient's insurance coverage and eligibility. Ensure that all necessary patient demographic information, such as name, date of birth, address, and insurance details, is accurately collected and documented. This information is vital for proper claim submission.

2. Coding Accuracy and Compliance:

Assign accurate and compliant codes to each service provided using the appropriate coding systems (e.g., CPT, ICD, HCPCS). Ensure that coding adheres to coding guidelines and payer-specific requirements. Accurate coding is critical for appropriate reimbursement and reduces the risk of claim denials or audits.

3. Timely Claim Submission:

Submit claims in a timely manner, adhering to payer-specific deadlines. Prompt claim submission helps expedite reimbursement and minimizes delays in the revenue cycle. Familiarize yourself with each payer's submission timeline and ensure claims are submitted within the specified timeframes.

4. Electronic Claims Submission:

Utilize electronic claims submission whenever possible. Electronic claim submission is more efficient, reduces errors, and expedites the claims process. Use electronic data interchange (EDI) or practice management systems to transmit claims securely to payers.

5. Claim Form Completion:

When submitting paper claims, accurately complete the required claim forms, such as the CMS-1500 (for professional services) or UB-04 (for institutional services). Follow payer-specific guidelines for completing the claim forms, including information on coding, patient demographics, and supporting documentation.

6. Attach Supporting Documentation:

Include any necessary supporting documentation with the claim, such as medical records, operative reports, or other required documentation. Ensure that the documentation supports the services billed and helps validate the medical necessity of the procedures or treatments rendered.

7. Clean Claims:

Submit clean claims that meet all the necessary requirements and are free from errors or omissions. Clean claims have a higher likelihood of being processed quickly and accurately, reducing the potential for claim denials or payment delays.

8. Claim Tracking and Follow-up:

Establish a system for tracking claims to ensure they are received and processed by payers. Monitor the status of submitted claims and proactively follow up on any delayed or denied claims. Promptly address any claim issues, resubmitting or appealing claims when necessary.

9. Payer-Specific Requirements:

Familiarize yourself with payer-specific requirements, such as preferred coding methodologies, modifiers, and documentation requirements. Each payer may have unique guidelines, coverage policies, and billing rules that must be followed for successful claims submission.

10. Claim Submission Compliance:

Ensure compliance with all applicable laws, regulations, and payer policies when submitting claims. Familiarize yourself with the billing and coding compliance requirements, including fraud and abuse regulations, anti-kickback laws, and HIPAA privacy and security regulations.

11. Claims Reconciliation:

Reconcile remittance advice (RA) or Explanation of Benefits (EOB) received from payers with the original claim submissions. Verify that the reimbursement amounts and payment details align with the services billed. Identify and resolve any discrepancies or underpayments to ensure accurate revenue recognition.

By following these key considerations and payer-specific requirements, healthcare organizations can streamline the claims submission process, minimize claim denials, and optimize revenue cycle management. Regularly monitor and analyze claims data to identify trends, address potential issues, and continuously improve the claims submission process.

Submitting clean claims is essential for efficient claims processing, timely reimbursement, and minimizing claim denials. Clean claims are those that meet all the necessary requirements and have a higher likelihood of being processed accurately by payers. Here are key principles and best practices for ensuring clean claims submission:

1. Accuracy in Documentation and Coding:

Ensure accurate and complete documentation of the services provided and assign appropriate codes based on the documentation. Adhere to coding guidelines, use standardized terminology, and capture the specificity and details necessary for accurate code assignment.

2. Verification of Patient and Insurance Information:

Verify patient demographic information, insurance coverage, and eligibility before submitting the claim. Ensure accurate entry of patient details, including name, date of birth, address, and insurance policy information. Confirm the accuracy of insurance information to avoid claim rejections.

3. Adherence to Coding and Billing Guidelines:

Follow coding and billing guidelines established by coding authorities and payers. Stay updated with changes in coding rules, payer-specific guidelines, and billing regulations. Adhering to these guidelines ensures compliance and reduces the risk of claim denials.

4. Timely Claims Submission:

Submit claims within the specified timelines outlined by payers. Familiarize yourself with each payer's submission deadlines and ensure claims are submitted promptly. Late submissions can lead to delayed reimbursement or claim denials.

5. Utilization of Electronic Claims Submission:

Utilize electronic claims submission whenever possible. Electronic claims are more accurate and efficient than paper claims, reducing the chances of errors and facilitating faster processing. Use electronic data interchange (EDI) or practice management systems to submit claims electronically.

6. Complete and Accurate Claim Forms:

When submitting paper claims, accurately complete the required claim forms, such as the CMS-1500 (for professional services) or UB-04 (for institutional services). Ensure all mandatory fields are completed, and information is entered accurately, legibly, and without errors.

7. Attachment of Supporting Documentation:

Include any necessary supporting documentation with the claim submission. Attach relevant medical records, operative reports, or other required documentation that supports the services billed. Proper documentation strengthens the claim's validity and helps justify the medical necessity of the services provided.

8. Review and Verification:

Review claims for accuracy, completeness, and adherence to payer-specific requirements before submission. Double-check the entered codes, patient information, and supporting documentation to minimize errors and omissions. Verify that all required fields are completed accurately.

9. Claims Tracking and Follow-up:

Implement a system for tracking claims throughout the entire claims process. Monitor the status of submitted claims, including acknowledgment of receipt by the payer and the processing timeline. Proactively follow up on any delayed or denied claims, resubmitting or appealing claims when necessary.

10. Compliance with Regulations:

Ensure compliance with all applicable laws, regulations, and payer policies when submitting claims. Familiarize yourself with billing and coding compliance requirements, including fraud and abuse regulations, anti-kickback laws, and HIPAA privacy and security regulations.

11. Continuous Process Improvement:

Regularly analyze claim submission data, identify trends, and address any recurring issues. Implement continuous process improvement initiatives to streamline the claims submission process, reduce errors, and enhance efficiency in revenue cycle management.

By adhering to these clean claim principles and best practices, healthcare organizations can improve their claims acceptance rates, reduce claim denials, and accelerate reimbursement. Clean claims promote efficient revenue cycle management, minimize revenue leakage, and contribute to financial stability within healthcare organizations.

Payer adjudication refers to the process by which payers review and evaluate submitted claims to determine the appropriate reimbursement. Claim rejection occurs when a claim is not accepted by the payer due to errors, missing information, or non-compliance with payer-specific guidelines. Analyzing payer adjudication and claim rejections helps identify common issues, address root causes, and improve revenue cycle management. Here are key considerations for payer adjudication and claim rejection analysis:

1. Claim Rejection Analysis:

Conduct a thorough analysis of claim rejections to identify patterns, trends, and common reasons for claim denials. Categorize claim rejection reasons, such as coding errors, missing documentation, eligibility issues, or non-covered services. Use claims management software or reporting tools to generate reports for analysis.

2. Payer-Specific Guidelines:

Understand and comply with payer-specific guidelines, coverage policies, and billing rules. Familiarize yourself with each payer's requirements, coding preferences, and documentation criteria. Analyze claim rejections related to non-compliance with payer guidelines and address any knowledge gaps or training needs.

3. Coding Accuracy and Compliance:

Review claim rejections related to coding errors or non-compliant coding practices. Assess the accuracy of code assignment, documentation, and adherence to coding guidelines. Provide education and training to coding professionals and healthcare providers to improve coding accuracy and compliance.

4. Documentation Deficiencies:

Analyze claim rejections due to missing or incomplete documentation. Identify areas where documentation can be improved to support the medical necessity and appropriateness of services provided. Enhance communication and collaboration between healthcare providers and coders to ensure comprehensive and accurate documentation.

5. Eligibility Verification:

Review claim rejections related to eligibility issues. Assess the effectiveness of the patient and insurance verification process to ensure accurate eligibility checks before claim submission. Implement automated eligibility verification tools or integrate with payer systems to minimize eligibility-related claim rejections.

6. Denial Management Process:

Evaluate the denial management process to identify opportunities for improvement. Analyze the effectiveness of denial tracking, follow-up, and appeals processes. Develop strategies to streamline and expedite the resolution of claim rejections, including proactive communication with payers and timely resubmission of corrected claims.

7. Timeliness of Claim Submission:

Analyze claim rejections related to late submissions or missed deadlines. Review the claim submission process to ensure timely claim submissions according to payer-specific timelines. Implement reminders and monitoring systems to avoid delayed claim submissions.

8. Communication with Payers:

Assess the effectiveness of communication channels with payers regarding claim rejections. Evaluate the clarity and completeness of claim resubmission communications and any required documentation. Establish open lines of communication with payers to resolve claim rejections efficiently and address any ongoing issues.

9. Staff Education and Training:

Provide ongoing education and training to staff members involved in the claims submission process. Keep them updated with coding and billing changes, payer requirements, and best practices. Continuously train staff on the proper interpretation of payer guidelines and compliance with billing regulations.

10. Performance Monitoring and KPIs:

Establish key performance indicators (KPIs) to monitor claim rejection rates, denial turnaround time, and appeals success rate. Regularly track and analyze these metrics to evaluate the effectiveness of denial management strategies and identify areas for improvement.

By analyzing payer adjudication and claim rejections, healthcare organizations can identify process inefficiencies, coding errors, and documentation gaps that contribute to claim denials. Implementing improvements based on the analysis findings can optimize revenue cycle management, reduce claim rejections, and increase reimbursement rates. Continuous monitoring and evaluation of payer adjudication and claim rejection data help drive ongoing process improvement and enhance financial performance.

Exercise 8: Claims Submission and Adjudication

1. Claims Submission Process and Requirements

Question 1: What is the purpose of the claims submission process in revenue cycle management (RCM)?

Answer: The purpose of the claims submission process in RCM is to request reimbursement from insurance payers for healthcare services provided to patients. It involves submitting a claim that contains detailed information about the patient, the services rendered, and the associated charges. The claims submission process is essential for healthcare organizations to receive timely and accurate reimbursement for their services.

Question 2: What are some key requirements for a successful claims submission?

Answer: Some key requirements for a successful claims submission include:

- Complete and accurate patient and insurance information, including demographics, policy numbers, and coverage details.

- Proper coding of diagnoses and procedures using the appropriate code sets (CPT, ICD, HCPCS) based on the documentation.

- Supporting documentation, such as medical records, progress notes, and consent forms, as required by the payer.

- Compliance with coding and billing guidelines and regulations set by payers and regulatory bodies.

- Timely submission within the payer's specified timeframe to avoid claim denials or late submission penalties.

2. Clean Claim Principles and Best Practices

Question 1: What is a clean claim, and why is it important in revenue cycle management (RCM)?

Answer: A clean claim is a claim that is accurately completed and contains all the necessary information required for processing and reimbursement by the payer. It adheres to the payer's requirements and guidelines, resulting in a higher likelihood of timely and accurate payment. Clean claims are important in RCM because:

- They reduce the risk of claim denials, rejections, or delays in payment.

- They streamline the claims adjudication process, allowing for faster reimbursement.

- They minimize the need for manual intervention or additional documentation requests from the payer.

- They improve overall operational efficiency by reducing the need for claim rework or resubmission.

Question 2: What are some best practices for ensuring clean claims submission?

Answer: Some best practices for ensuring clean claims submission include:

- Utilizing electronic claims submission whenever possible, as it reduces errors and speeds up processing.

- Implementing claims scrubbing software or tools that can perform automated checks for errors or missing information before submission.

- Conducting regular audits and quality checks on claims data and documentation to identify and address any issues or discrepancies.

- Training and educating staff on proper coding, documentation, and claims submission processes to ensure consistency and accuracy.

- Staying updated with payer-specific requirements and guidelines to ensure compliance and avoid common pitfalls.

- Establishing effective communication channels with payers to clarify any unclear or ambiguous guidelines and resolve issues promptly.

3. Payer Adjudication and Claim Rejection Analysis

Question 1: What is payer adjudication in the claims process, and why is it important?

Answer: Payer adjudication is the process by which insurance payers review and evaluate submitted claims to determine the reimbursement amount based on the patient's insurance coverage, policy terms, and agreed-upon payment rates. It involves assessing the claim's validity, checking for coding accuracy, and applying the payer's reimbursement methodologies and policies. Payer adjudication is important because:

- It determines the amount of reimbursement healthcare organizations receive for the services provided.

- It ensures that claims are processed and paid accurately and in compliance with contractual agreements and regulatory guidelines.

- It helps identify and address any discrepancies or issues in coding, documentation, or reimbursement that may require further action or clarification.

- It provides an opportunity for healthcare organizations to appeal or address claim denials or underpayments, ensuring proper reimbursement.

Question 2: What is the significance of claim rejection analysis in revenue cycle management (RCM)?

Answer: Claim rejection analysis is significant in RCM because it allows healthcare organizations to identify and address the reasons for claim rejections or denials. By analyzing rejected claims, organizations can:

- Identify patterns or common issues that lead to claim rejections, such as coding errors, missing documentation, or non-compliance with payer guidelines.

- Take corrective actions, such as providing additional documentation, correcting coding errors, or appealing claim denials, to ensure proper reimbursement.

- Improve operational efficiency by addressing root causes of claim rejections and implementing process improvements or staff training to prevent future rejections.

- Maximize revenue potential by minimizing claim denials and optimizing reimbursement rates.

- Strengthen relationships with payers by resolving claim-related issues promptly and maintaining a smooth claims submission and adjudication process.

These exercises provide an opportunity to reinforce the knowledge gained from the chapter on Claims Submission and Adjudication. The questions assess understanding and reinforce key concepts related to the claims submission process and requirements, clean claim principles and best practices, and payer adjudication and claim rejection analysis in revenue cycle management.

9. Denial Management and Appeals

9.1 Understanding Claim Denials and Common Causes:

Claim denials occur when a submitted claim is not reimbursed by the payer due to various reasons. Understanding the common causes of claim denials is crucial for effective denial management and appeals. Here are key considerations for understanding claim denials and their common causes:

1. Definition of Claim Denial:

A claim denial is the refusal of a payer to reimburse a submitted claim, either partially or entirely, for healthcare services rendered. Denials can occur for a variety of reasons, including coding errors, missing or incomplete documentation, eligibility issues, non-covered services, and non-compliance with payer-specific guidelines.

2. Common Causes of Claim Denials:

While claim denials can be attributed to various factors, here are some common causes:

a. Coding Errors: Inaccurate or non-compliant coding, such as incorrect procedure codes, modifiers, or diagnosis codes, can lead to claim denials. This may include unbundling or incorrect use of modifiers, insufficient documentation to support the codes assigned, or mismatched codes and procedures.

b. Missing or Incomplete Documentation: Claims can be denied if the documentation fails to support the medical necessity of the services provided or lacks essential information required by the payer. Insufficient documentation, missing signatures, or incomplete patient information can result in claim denials.

c. Eligibility and Coverage Issues: Claim denials can occur when the patient's insurance coverage is not active, the service provided is not covered under the policy, or there are limitations or exclusions related to the service rendered. Failure to verify patient eligibility or pre-authorization requirements can lead to denials.

d. Timeliness and Filing Errors: Claims submitted beyond the payer's specified deadline or with errors in the claim form, such as missing or incorrect patient information, can be denied. Late submissions and filing errors can result in claim denials or payment delays.

e. Medical Necessity and Documentation Requirements: Payers may deny claims if they determine that the services provided were not medically necessary or lacked appropriate documentation to support the level of care. Failure to meet documentation requirements or provide sufficient justification for the services rendered can result in denials.

f. Coordination of Benefits (COB) Issues: In cases where the patient has multiple insurance coverages, claim denials can occur due to coordination of benefits errors, such as incorrect primary/secondary payer information or lack of coordination between payers.

g. Payer Policy and Reimbursement Changes: Denials can result from changes in payer policies, reimbursement rates, or coverage guidelines. Failure to stay updated with payer policy changes and adjust billing practices accordingly can lead to claim denials.

h. Administrative and Data Entry Errors: Mistakes in claim data entry, such as typographical errors, incorrect patient information, or transposed digits, can result in claim denials. Accuracy in data entry and claim submission is essential to avoid administrative errors.

3. Importance of Denial Analysis:

Analyzing claim denials is crucial for identifying patterns, trends, and root causes. By conducting a thorough denial analysis, healthcare organizations can pinpoint recurring issues, implement corrective actions, and improve revenue cycle management. Denial analysis helps optimize coding accuracy, enhance documentation practices, and identify opportunities for staff education and training.

4. Prevention and Denial Management Strategies:

Implement proactive denial management strategies to minimize claim denials. This includes:

a. Education and Training: Provide ongoing education and training to coding professionals, billing staff, and healthcare providers to ensure accurate coding, proper documentation practices, and compliance with payer guidelines.

b. Coding Audits: Conduct regular coding audits to identify coding errors and deficiencies. Address coding discrepancies through targeted education, process improvements, and monitoring.

c. Documentation Improvement: Enhance documentation practices to ensure comprehensive, accurate, and compliant documentation. Emphasize the importance of complete and detailed documentation that supports the medical necessity of services provided.

d. Eligibility Verification: Implement robust processes for verifying patient eligibility and coverage. Verify insurance information, pre-authorization requirements, and coverage limitations to minimize denials related to eligibility issues.

e. Claim Scrubbing: Utilize claim scrubbing tools or software that perform automated checks to identify potential errors, coding issues, and missing information before claim submission. This helps reduce denials related to data entry errors and coding inaccuracies.

f. Appeals Process: Develop an effective appeals process to challenge claim denials. Timely follow up on denied claims, gather supporting documentation, and submit appeals with clear explanations and justification for reimbursement.

g. Payer Communication: Establish open lines of communication with payers to address claim denials promptly. Engage in proactive dialogue, seek clarification on denial reasons, and resolve issues through effective communication and negotiation.

h. Performance Monitoring: Continuously monitor denial rates, denial reasons, and appeals success rates to gauge the effectiveness of denial management strategies. Identify areas for improvement and implement targeted interventions.

By understanding the common causes of claim denials and implementing proactive denial management strategies, healthcare organizations can reduce claim denials, improve revenue cycle performance, and optimize reimbursement. Regular denial analysis and continuous process improvement are essential for effective denial management and appeals.

9.2 Denial Prevention and Resolution Strategies:

Denial prevention and resolution strategies are essential for effective revenue cycle management. By implementing proactive measures to prevent denials and employing effective strategies to resolve denied claims, healthcare organizations can optimize reimbursement and minimize revenue leakage. Here are key strategies for denial prevention and resolution:

1. Education and Training:

Provide comprehensive education and training to coding professionals, billing staff, and healthcare providers on coding guidelines, documentation requirements, and payer policies. Ongoing training ensures a thorough understanding of the billing process and helps prevent coding errors and documentation deficiencies.

2. Coding Accuracy and Compliance:

Emphasize the importance of accurate and compliant coding practices. Conduct regular coding audits to identify coding errors and address any discrepancies. Ensure coding professionals stay updated with the latest coding guidelines and regulations to minimize coding-related denials.

3. Documentation Improvement:

Enhance documentation practices to support the medical necessity of services rendered. Encourage providers to document all relevant information, including diagnoses, treatments, and patient progress. Improve communication between healthcare providers and coders to ensure complete and accurate documentation.

4. Eligibility Verification:

Implement robust processes for verifying patient eligibility and coverage prior to providing services. Verify insurance information, pre-authorization requirements, and coverage limitations to minimize denials related to eligibility issues. Regularly communicate with patients to update insurance information as needed.

5. Clear and Concise Communication:

Foster clear and concise communication with payers to reduce claim denials. Ensure accurate and complete claim submission with all required documentation and supporting information. Utilize standardized communication channels and follow payer-specific guidelines for claim submission.

6. Claim Scrubbing and Pre-Submission Checks:

Utilize claim scrubbing tools or software to identify potential errors, coding issues, and missing information before claim submission. Perform pre-submission checks to verify claim accuracy, coding compliance, and completeness. Correct any identified errors or discrepancies prior to claim submission.

7. Timely Claim Submission:

Adhere to payer-specific deadlines and submit claims in a timely manner. Monitor claim submission timelines and ensure claims are submitted promptly to avoid denials due to late submissions. Implement reminders and monitoring systems to facilitate timely claim submission.

8. Denial Analysis and Trend Identification:

Conduct thorough analysis of denied claims to identify patterns, trends, and root causes. Analyze denial data to pinpoint recurring issues and implement corrective actions. Use denial analysis to identify opportunities for process improvements, staff education, and training.

9. Effective Appeals Management:

Establish a robust appeals management process to challenge claim denials. Timely follow up on denied claims, gather supporting documentation, and submit appeals with clear explanations and justification for reimbursement. Track and monitor the progress of appeals to ensure timely resolution.

10. Collaboration with Payers:

Foster collaborative relationships with payers to resolve claim denials. Engage in proactive dialogue, seek clarification on denial reasons, and work collaboratively to address denials. Establish dedicated points of contact and open lines of communication to facilitate prompt resolution.

11. Performance Monitoring and Process Improvement:

Continuously monitor denial rates, denial reasons, appeals success rates, and other key performance indicators. Identify areas for improvement and implement targeted interventions. Regularly assess denial prevention and resolution strategies to drive process improvement and optimize revenue cycle performance.

By implementing these denial prevention and resolution strategies, healthcare organizations can proactively minimize claim denials, improve cash flow, and optimize reimbursement. Regular analysis, process refinement, and collaboration with payers contribute to effective denial management and revenue cycle success.

9.3 Effective Appeal Process and Maximizing Reimbursement:

An effective appeal process is essential for resolving denied claims and maximizing reimbursement in revenue cycle management. By following a structured approach and employing strategies to support appeals, healthcare organizations can increase their chances of successful appeals and optimize revenue. Here are key considerations for an effective appeal process and maximizing reimbursement:

1. Understand the Denial Reason:

Analyze the denial reason provided by the payer and thoroughly understand the basis for the claim denial. Review the denial letter or explanation of benefits (EOB) to identify specific issues or discrepancies that need to be addressed in the appeal.

2. Timely Appeals Submission:

Adhere to the payer's specified timelines for submitting appeals. Ensure appeals are submitted within the allotted timeframe to avoid potential claim rejection due to late submission. Establish internal processes and reminders to track and meet appeal submission deadlines.

3. Gather Supporting Documentation:

Collect all relevant supporting documentation to strengthen the appeal. This may include medical records, progress notes, operative reports, test results, and any other documentation that validates the medical necessity and appropriateness of the services provided. Ensure the documentation clearly supports the services billed and addresses the specific denial reason.

4. Prepare a Persuasive Appeal Letter:

Craft a well-structured and persuasive appeal letter that provides a clear explanation of the situation, addresses the denial reason, and presents compelling arguments supported by the collected documentation. Clearly state the case for reconsideration, citing applicable coding guidelines, payer policies, and medical necessity.

5. Know Payer Appeal Requirements:

Familiarize yourself with the payer's appeal requirements and guidelines. Understand the preferred mode of submission (e.g., online portal, fax, mail), any specific forms to be completed, and any additional information or documentation that must be included in the appeal package. Adhere to these requirements to ensure the appeal is processed without delays.

6. Utilize Payer Resources:

Utilize any available resources provided by the payer to support the appeal process. This may include contacting the payer's customer service or provider relations department to seek guidance on the appeal process, specific documentation requirements, or any additional information that may be helpful for a successful appeal.

7. Seek Expert Opinion:

Consult with coding experts, physician advisors, or legal counsel, if necessary, to strengthen the appeal case. Their expertise can provide valuable insights, help navigate complex coding or documentation issues, and increase the chances of a successful appeal.

8. Track and Monitor Appeals:

Establish a tracking system to monitor the status and progress of each appeal. Keep a record of all appeals submitted, including dates, details, and any correspondence or communication with the payer. Regularly follow up with the payer to check the status of the appeal and ensure it is being actively processed.

9. Analyze Appeals Outcomes:

Analyze the outcomes of appeals to identify trends and patterns. Evaluate the success rates, reasons for overturned denials, and any lessons learned from the appeal process. Use this analysis to improve internal processes, identify opportunities for education or training, and refine strategies to maximize reimbursement.

10. Continuous Process Improvement:

Continuously assess and refine the appeal process based on feedback, denials trends, and industry updates. Stay informed about coding changes, payer policies, and regulatory updates to adapt appeal strategies accordingly. Implement ongoing staff education and training to enhance coding accuracy and documentation practices.

11. Negotiation and Settlement:

In certain cases, negotiation or settlement may be an option to resolve denied claims. Engage in discussions with payers to explore potential resolutions, such as partial payment or alternative arrangements, that can mutually benefit both parties.

By following these strategies for an effective appeal process and implementing a proactive approach to maximize reimbursement, healthcare organizations can increase their success rates in appeals, optimize revenue recovery, and enhance revenue cycle management. Effective appeals management ensures that rightful reimbursement is obtained for services rendered, contributing to financial stability and viability.

Exercise 9: Denial Management and Appeals

1. Understanding Claim Denials and Common Causes

Question 1: What is a claim denial, and why do claim denials occur in the revenue cycle management (RCM) process?

Answer: A claim denial is the refusal of an insurance payer to reimburse a healthcare organization for a submitted claim. Claim denials can occur in the RCM process for various reasons, such as:

- Coding errors: Incorrect or incomplete coding, such as using the wrong codes or modifiers, can result in claim denials.

- Documentation deficiencies: Insufficient or missing documentation to support medical necessity or the services provided can lead to claim denials.

- Eligibility and coverage issues: Claim denials can occur if the patient's insurance coverage is inactive, the services are not covered, or prior authorization requirements are not met.

- Billing errors: Inaccurate billing, such as duplicate charges, incorrect dates, or mismatched patient and insurance information, can result in claim denials.

- Non-compliance with payer policies: Failure to adhere to specific payer guidelines, such as timely filing limits or utilization management requirements, can lead to claim denials.

Question 2: What are some common causes of claim denials in the RCM process?

Answer: Some common causes of claim denials in the RCM process include:

- Coding errors or omissions

- Insufficient or missing documentation

- Incorrect patient or insurance information

- Lack of prior authorization

- Incomplete or inaccurate claim submission

- Non-covered services or experimental procedures

- Timely filing limit exceeded

- Coordination of benefits issues

- Medical necessity not established

- Billing for services not rendered

2. Denial Prevention and Resolution Strategies

Question 1: What are some strategies for preventing claim denials in the revenue cycle management (RCM) process?

Answer: Strategies for preventing claim denials in the RCM process include:

- Ensuring accurate and complete documentation to support the services provided and medical necessity.

- Conducting regular coding and billing audits to identify and address coding errors, documentation deficiencies, and billing discrepancies.

- Verifying patient eligibility and insurance coverage before providing services and addressing any coverage limitations or prior authorization requirements.

- Implementing electronic claims submission and utilizing claims scrubbing software to catch errors before submission.

- Training and educating staff on coding guidelines, documentation requirements, and payer policies to ensure compliance and accuracy.

- Establishing effective communication channels with payers to clarify any ambiguous guidelines or resolve issues promptly.

- Implementing denial management software or systems to track and analyze denial trends and proactively address common causes.

Question 2: What are some strategies for effectively resolving claim denials in the RCM process?

Answer: Strategies for effectively resolving claim denials in the RCM process include:

- Reviewing the denial reason and determining the appropriate course of action, such as resubmitting the claim, appealing the denial, or correcting errors and resubmitting.

- Gathering any additional documentation or information needed to support the claim and address the reason for denial.

- Following the payer's guidelines and requirements for filing appeals, including submitting appeals within the specified timeframe.

- Providing clear and concise explanations in the appeal, addressing the denial reason and providing supporting documentation or evidence.

- Monitoring the status of appeals and following up with payers to ensure timely resolution.

- Analyzing denial patterns and trends to identify opportunities for process improvement and proactive prevention of future denials.

- Collaborating with clinical and administrative staff to address root causes of denials and implement changes to prevent similar denials in the future.

3. Effective Appeal Process and Maximizing Reimbursement

Question 1: What is the purpose of the appeal process in the revenue cycle management (RCM) process?

Answer: The purpose of the appeal process in RCM is to challenge a claim denial and request reconsideration or reversal of the decision by the insurance payer. The appeal process is an opportunity for healthcare organizations to provide additional information, clarify any misunderstandings, and advocate for proper reimbursement. It aims to maximize reimbursement by addressing claim denials and ensuring that the organization receives fair and accurate payment for services rendered.

Question 2: What are some key considerations for an effective appeal process in RCM?

Answer: Some key considerations for an effective appeal process in RCM include:

- Familiarizing oneself with the payer's appeal guidelines, requirements, and timelines.

- Reviewing the denial reason and gathering all necessary documentation and supporting evidence to address the denial.

- Composing a well-written appeal letter that clearly explains the reason for the appeal, provides supporting documentation, and addresses any specific points raised by the payer in the denial.

- Submitting the appeal within the specified timeframe and following any specific submission requirements or formats.

- Keeping detailed records of all communication and documentation related to the appeal.

- Monitoring the status of the appeal and following up with the payer if necessary.

- Analyzing the outcomes of appeals to identify trends, areas for improvement, and opportunities to enhance denial prevention strategies.

These exercises provide an opportunity to reinforce the knowledge gained from the chapter on Denial Management and Appeals. The questions assess understanding and reinforce key concepts related to understanding claim denials and their common causes, strategies for denial prevention and resolution, and the effective appeal process for maximizing reimbursement in revenue cycle management.

10. Insurance Follow-Up and Accounts Receivable Management

10.1 Monitoring Unpaid Claims and Aging Reports:

Monitoring unpaid claims and aging reports is crucial for effective insurance follow-up and accounts receivable management. It helps identify outstanding claims, track payment delays, and take necessary actions to ensure timely reimbursement. Here are key considerations for monitoring unpaid claims and aging reports:

1. Unpaid Claims Management:

Regularly review the status of submitted claims to identify unpaid or outstanding claims. Track claims from the date of submission to the date of payment or denial. Implement a system to monitor claims throughout the entire claims lifecycle and ensure timely follow-up.

2. Aging Reports:

Generate and analyze aging reports that provide a snapshot of the unpaid claims based on the duration since submission. Aging reports categorize claims into different time periods (e.g., 30 days, 60 days, 90 days, etc.) to highlight the aging of unpaid claims. These reports help prioritize follow-up efforts and identify claims that require immediate attention.

3. Claim Reconciliation:

Reconcile remittance advice (RA) or Explanation of Benefits (EOB) received from payers with the original claim submissions. Verify that payments align with the expected reimbursement amounts and reconcile any discrepancies. Promptly address underpayments, denials, or any other issues identified during the reconciliation process.

4. Follow-Up Process:

Establish a systematic follow-up process for unpaid claims. Assign dedicated staff members or teams responsible for monitoring unpaid claims and initiating follow-up actions. Implement reminders and task management systems to ensure timely follow-up calls, emails, or other forms of communication with payers.

5. Communication with Payers:

Maintain open lines of communication with payers to resolve claim payment issues. Proactively reach out to payers to inquire about the status of unpaid claims, confirm receipt of claims, or seek clarification on any outstanding issues. Document all communications and follow-up actions taken for future reference.

6. Claim Resubmission and Appeals:

Identify claims that require resubmission or appeals due to denials or payment discrepancies. Determine the appropriate action based on the denial reason and supporting documentation. Follow the payer's guidelines for resubmission or appeals to maximize the chances of successful resolution.

7. Denial Trend Analysis:

Analyze claim denial trends to identify recurring issues and root causes. Identify patterns or common reasons for denials, such as coding errors, documentation deficiencies, or eligibility issues. Use this analysis to address the underlying issues, implement process improvements, and enhance staff training and education.

8. Timely Filing Compliance:

Ensure compliance with payer-specific timely filing requirements. Monitor aging reports to identify claims approaching the filing deadlines and take prompt action to prevent potential denials due to late filing. Familiarize yourself with each payer's specific timely filing guidelines and implement internal processes to meet the deadlines.

9. Accounts Receivable Aging Analysis:

Conduct a comprehensive analysis of accounts receivable aging reports to assess the overall financial health of the organization. Evaluate the distribution of outstanding claims across different aging categories and identify areas of concern. Implement strategies to reduce the aging of accounts receivable and expedite the collection of outstanding payments.

10. Performance Monitoring and Metrics:

Establish key performance indicators (KPIs) to monitor the effectiveness of insurance follow-up and accounts receivable management. Track metrics such as claim turnaround time, average days in accounts receivable, denial rates, and collection rates. Regularly analyze these metrics to evaluate performance, identify bottlenecks, and implement targeted interventions for improvement.

By diligently monitoring unpaid claims and aging reports, healthcare organizations can proactively manage their accounts receivable, optimize revenue cycle performance, and ensure timely reimbursement.

Effective insurance follow-up and accounts receivable management contribute to financial stability and the overall success of the organization.

10.2 Timely and Effective Follow-Up Strategies:

Timely and effective follow-up strategies are essential for managing unpaid claims and maximizing reimbursement. Implementing structured processes and employing proactive follow-up strategies can expedite claim resolution and improve revenue cycle management. Here are key strategies for timely and effective follow-up:

1. Establish Clear Follow-Up Guidelines:

Develop clear guidelines and protocols for follow-up activities. Define specific timelines for initial follow-up after claim submission and subsequent follow-up intervals based on payer-specific guidelines. Document these guidelines to ensure consistency and accountability among staff members responsible for follow-up.

2. Prioritize Unpaid Claims:

Prioritize unpaid claims based on factors such as the aging of the claim, the dollar amount, or the payer's payment patterns. Focus on high-value claims, those approaching timely filing deadlines, or claims with recurring denials. Prioritization helps allocate resources effectively and ensure timely resolution for critical claims.

3. Automation and Technology:

Leverage technology solutions, such as practice management systems or revenue cycle management software, to automate follow-up activities. Utilize features like claims tracking, task management, and reminders to streamline follow-up processes and ensure timely actions. Automation reduces manual efforts, minimizes errors, and improves efficiency.

4. Regularly Review Aging Reports:

Review aging reports on a regular basis to identify unpaid claims that require follow-up. Analyze aging reports by payer, aging category, or other relevant criteria to prioritize follow-up efforts. Set a schedule for reviewing aging reports to ensure consistent monitoring of unpaid claims.

5. Utilize Electronic Tools and Portals:

Take advantage of electronic tools and payer portals for claim status inquiries and follow-up. Many payers offer online portals or electronic tools that provide real-time claim status updates. Utilize these resources to track claim progress, check payment details, and communicate directly with payers.

6. Proactive Communication:

Initiate proactive communication with payers to inquire about claim status or resolve outstanding issues. Contact payers via phone, email, or payer-specific online communication channels. Clearly articulate the purpose of communication, provide necessary details, and document all conversations for future reference.

7. Appeal and Resubmission Management:

Develop a systematic approach for managing claim appeals and resubmissions. Ensure appeals are submitted within the specified timelines and include all relevant documentation and supporting information. Track the progress of appeals and resubmissions, following up with payers as needed to expedite resolution.

8. Escalation Procedures:

Establish escalation procedures for unresolved or long-pending claims. Define criteria for escalating claims to higher levels within the payer's organization or engaging in dispute resolution processes. Ensure clear lines of communication and defined escalation paths to escalate unresolved claims appropriately.

9. Staff Training and Education:

Provide ongoing training and education to staff members responsible for follow-up activities. Keep them updated on payer-specific guidelines, coding changes, and industry best practices. Enhance their knowledge and skills in effective communication, negotiation, and problem-solving to facilitate successful follow-up.

10. Performance Monitoring and Analysis:

Regularly monitor and analyze follow-up performance metrics, such as average days in accounts receivable, claim resolution rates, and collection rates. Identify trends, areas of improvement, and potential bottlenecks. Use these insights to refine follow-up strategies, enhance processes, and optimize revenue cycle management.

11. Continuous Process Improvement:

Foster a culture of continuous improvement in follow-up processes. Encourage feedback from staff members involved in follow-up activities, gather suggestions for process enhancements, and implement changes based on identified opportunities. Regularly assess and refine follow-up strategies to drive efficiency and productivity.

By implementing these timely and effective follow-up strategies, healthcare organizations can streamline claims resolution, accelerate reimbursement, and enhance overall revenue cycle performance. Proactive and diligent follow-up practices contribute to improved cash flow, reduced accounts receivable aging, and increased financial stability.

10.3 Reducing Days in Accounts Receivable (DAR):

Reducing Days in Accounts Receivable (DAR) is a critical goal in revenue cycle management. It represents the average number of days it takes for a healthcare organization to collect payments from insurance companies and patients. A lower DAR indicates a more efficient revenue cycle and faster cash flow. Here are key strategies to reduce DAR:

1. Streamline Claims Submission:

Optimize the claims submission process to minimize delays. Ensure accurate and complete claim information, including coding, documentation, and supporting documents. Leverage electronic claims submission whenever possible to expedite the process and reduce manual errors.

2. Verify Eligibility and Coverage:

Verify patient eligibility and insurance coverage before providing services. Confirm insurance information, pre-authorization requirements, and coverage limitations. Avoid rendering services that may not be covered, reducing the risk of claim denials and payment delays.

3. Accurate and Compliant Coding:

Ensure accurate and compliant coding practices. Adhere to coding guidelines, use appropriate modifiers, and document services accurately. Proactive education and ongoing training for coding professionals can help reduce coding errors and subsequent claim rejections.

4. Prompt Claims Follow-up:

Establish a systematic process for claims follow-up. Regularly review aging reports to identify unpaid claims, and promptly follow up with payers to inquire about the status and resolve outstanding issues. Timely and proactive follow-up helps expedite claim resolution and payment.

5. Denial Management and Appeals:

Implement an effective denial management process to minimize claim denials. Analyze denial patterns, address root causes, and appeal denials when appropriate. Swift action in response to denials helps accelerate claim resolution and reduces the time spent in accounts receivable.

6. Implement Clear Payment Policies:

Establish clear and consistent payment policies for patients. Clearly communicate expectations regarding payment terms, insurance coverage, copayments, and deductibles. Offer convenient payment options, such as online portals or electronic payment systems, to facilitate prompt patient payments.

7. Enhance Patient Financial Counseling:

Provide comprehensive financial counseling to patients to ensure they understand their financial responsibilities. Offer assistance in understanding insurance coverage, explaining billing statements, and exploring financial assistance programs. This reduces payment delays and improves patient satisfaction.

8. Expedite Claim Reconciliation:

Streamline the claim reconciliation process to identify and address discrepancies efficiently. Regularly reconcile remittance advice or Explanation of Benefits (EOB) received from payers with the original claim submissions. Address underpayments or denials promptly to expedite correct payment.

9. Optimize Revenue Cycle Technology:

Leverage technology solutions, such as revenue cycle management software or practice management systems, to automate processes, streamline workflows, and track accounts receivable. Utilize features like automated claim status checks and reminders to minimize manual effort and expedite claim resolution.

10. Monitor Key Performance Indicators (KPIs):

Continuously monitor DAR and other key performance indicators related to accounts receivable. Regularly analyze data to identify trends, benchmark performance, and track progress. Set goals and targets for reducing DAR and hold regular performance review meetings to drive accountability.

11. Collaboration with Payers:

Foster collaborative relationships with payers to facilitate timely reimbursement. Engage in proactive communication, address payment issues promptly, and negotiate payment terms when necessary. Building strong relationships with payers can help expedite claims processing and reduce DAR.

12. Continuous Process Improvement:

Foster a culture of continuous improvement within the revenue cycle. Encourage staff members to provide feedback and suggestions for process enhancements. Regularly evaluate existing processes, identify areas for improvement, and implement changes to streamline operations and reduce DAR.

By implementing these strategies, healthcare organizations can reduce Days in Accounts Receivable (DAR), accelerate cash flow, and improve financial performance. A proactive and efficient revenue cycle management approach enhances overall operational efficiency and contributes to long-term sustainability.

Exercise 10: Insurance Follow-Up and Accounts Receivable Management

1. Monitoring Unpaid Claims and Aging Reports

Question 1: Why is it important for healthcare organizations to monitor unpaid claims and aging reports in revenue cycle management (RCM)?

Answer: It is important for healthcare organizations to monitor unpaid claims and aging reports in RCM because:

- It helps identify outstanding claims that require follow-up to ensure timely reimbursement.

- It allows organizations to track the aging of unpaid claims and prioritize follow-up based on the time elapsed since the claim was submitted.

- It helps identify trends or patterns in claim denials or delays, enabling targeted interventions to address common issues.

- It provides visibility into the financial health of the organization by tracking the amount and age of outstanding claims.

- It helps optimize cash flow by identifying and addressing bottlenecks in the reimbursement process.

Question 2: What is an aging report, and how does it assist in managing accounts receivable?

Answer: An aging report is a financial report that categorizes accounts receivable based on the length of time the claims have been outstanding. It typically breaks down outstanding claims into different age buckets, such as 30, 60, 90, or 120+ days. The aging report assists in managing accounts receivable by:

- Providing a snapshot of the organization's outstanding claims and their age distribution.

- Helping identify claims that require immediate attention or escalated follow-up due to prolonged aging.

- Enabling prioritization of follow-up activities based on the urgency of unpaid claims.

- Assisting in identifying trends or patterns in delayed payments or denials.

- Facilitating communication and collaboration among revenue cycle staff, providers, and payers to resolve outstanding claims.

2. Timely and Effective Follow-Up Strategies

Question 1: What are some strategies for conducting timely and effective follow-up on unpaid claims in revenue cycle management (RCM)?

Answer: Some strategies for conducting timely and effective follow-up on unpaid claims in RCM include:

- Establishing clear follow-up workflows and assigning responsibilities to specific staff members to ensure accountability.

- Utilizing technology tools, such as automated reminders and task management systems, to track and monitor follow-up activities.

- Setting specific follow-up timeframes based on payer requirements or industry benchmarks.

- Prioritizing follow-up based on the age, amount, or importance of unpaid claims.

- Conducting thorough research and investigation before contacting payers, ensuring all necessary information and documentation are available.

- Establishing effective communication channels with payers, such as designated contacts or provider portals, to streamline follow-up communication.

- Documenting all follow-up activities, including dates, contacts, and outcomes, to maintain a clear audit trail and ensure continuity of follow-up efforts.

Question 2: How can effective follow-up strategies contribute to improved accounts receivable management?

Answer: Effective follow-up strategies contribute to improved accounts receivable management by:

- Facilitating timely reimbursement and reducing the average number of days in accounts receivable (DAR).

- Identifying and resolving issues that may be causing delays or denials, leading to improved cash flow.

- Reducing the risk of claim write-offs or uncollectible accounts by proactively addressing unpaid claims.

- Enhancing payer-provider relationships by demonstrating proactive and efficient revenue cycle management practices.

- Increasing overall revenue by minimizing the amount of outstanding accounts receivable and optimizing reimbursement.

- Improving operational efficiency by streamlining follow-up processes, minimizing time spent on unproductive tasks, and maximizing staff productivity.

3. Reducing Days in Accounts Receivable (DAR)

Question 1: Why is reducing the number of days in accounts receivable (DAR) important for healthcare organizations?

Answer: Reducing the number of days in accounts receivable (DAR) is important for healthcare organizations because:

- It improves cash flow by shortening the time between providing services and receiving payment.

- It allows organizations to allocate financial resources more efficiently and meet their financial obligations promptly.

- It minimizes the risk of bad debt and write-offs by reducing the amount of uncollected accounts receivable.

- It provides financial stability and flexibility to invest in resources, technology, and growth opportunities.

- It improves the organization's financial performance and profitability by optimizing revenue collection and minimizing outstanding balances.

Question 2: What are some strategies for reducing days in accounts receivable (DAR) in revenue cycle management (RCM)?

Answer: Some strategies for reducing days in accounts receivable (DAR) in RCM include:

- Implementing efficient billing and claims submission processes to minimize delays and denials.

- Conducting timely and effective follow-up on unpaid claims to accelerate reimbursement.

- Implementing effective denial management strategies to address claim denials and prevent delayed payments.

- Offering convenient payment options and implementing patient-friendly billing practices to encourage timely payments.

- Streamlining and automating revenue cycle processes, such as eligibility verification and claims adjudication, to minimize manual errors and delays.

- Conducting regular audits and quality checks to identify and address issues that may contribute to delayed payments.

- Establishing strong relationships with payers through regular communication and collaboration to resolve outstanding issues promptly.

These exercises provide an opportunity to reinforce the knowledge gained from the chapter on Insurance Follow-Up and Accounts Receivable Management. The questions assess understanding and reinforce key concepts related to monitoring unpaid claims and aging reports, timely and effective follow-up strategies, and reducing days in accounts receivable (DAR) in revenue cycle management.

11. Patient Billing and Collections

11.1 Overview of Patient Billing Cycle:

The patient billing cycle encompasses the processes involved in generating and managing patient bills for healthcare services rendered. It includes activities such as creating and delivering accurate bills, explaining charges to patients, and collecting payments. Here's an overview of the patient billing cycle:

1. Patient Registration and Insurance Verification:

At the initial point of contact, patients provide their demographic and insurance information during the registration process. Insurance verification is performed to validate coverage, eligibility, and any pre-authorization requirements.

2. Service Documentation and Coding:

Healthcare providers document the services provided, diagnoses, and procedures performed during the patient visit. Accurate and compliant coding is applied to translate the services into standardized codes (CPT, ICD, HCPCS) for billing and reimbursement purposes.

3. Claim Generation and Submission:

Claims are generated based on the coded services and submitted to insurance payers for reimbursement. Claims may be submitted electronically or in paper form, depending on payer requirements. Timely submission is crucial to ensure prompt reimbursement.

4. Insurance Adjudication:

Insurance payers review and process the submitted claims. They assess the claims for coding accuracy, medical necessity, and adherence to payer-specific policies. The payer determines the reimbursement amount based on the contractual agreement with the healthcare provider.

5. Explanation of Benefits (EOB):

After the insurance payer processes the claim, an Explanation of Benefits (EOB) is generated. The EOB provides a detailed breakdown of the services billed, the allowed amount, the patient's financial responsibility, and any denial or adjustment information.

6. Patient Billing Statement:

A patient billing statement is created based on the EOB and the patient's financial responsibility. It includes a summary of charges, insurance payments, and any outstanding balance. The statement may also provide explanations and instructions for payment options.

7. Patient Education and Communication:

Healthcare organizations communicate with patients to explain the billing statement, answer questions, and clarify any concerns. This includes providing information about insurance coverage, co-pays, deductibles, and the payment process. Patient education regarding financial assistance programs and payment plans may also be provided.

8. Payment Collection:

Patients are responsible for paying their portion of the charges as indicated on the billing statement. Payment collection methods can include cash, checks, credit cards, and electronic funds transfers. Healthcare organizations may offer various payment options, such as online portals or payment plans, to facilitate timely payments.

9. Accounts Receivable Management:

Healthcare organizations monitor and manage outstanding patient balances through accounts receivable management. This involves tracking unpaid patient balances, sending reminders for overdue payments, and pursuing collections activities when necessary. Clear policies and procedures for managing accounts receivable are established to ensure consistent and efficient collection efforts.

10. Follow-Up and Resolution:

If a patient's account remains unpaid or in dispute, follow-up activities are initiated to address the outstanding balance. This may involve contacting the patient to resolve payment issues, offering payment arrangements, or engaging in negotiations for settlement. Timely and proactive follow-up helps minimize the aging of patient accounts receivable.

11. Financial Reporting and Analysis:

Regular financial reporting and analysis are conducted to monitor the effectiveness of the patient billing cycle. Key performance indicators (KPIs) such as average days in accounts receivable, collection rates, and aging of patient balances are tracked to evaluate performance and identify areas for improvement.

Efficient management of the patient billing cycle ensures accurate billing, prompt payment, and positive patient experiences. Healthcare organizations should implement clear communication, streamlined processes, and effective billing systems to optimize revenue cycle performance and maintain financial stability.

11.2 Clear and Transparent Patient Statements:

Clear and transparent patient statements are essential for effective communication, fostering patient understanding, and facilitating prompt payment. Providing patients with easily comprehensible billing statements helps build trust, reduces confusion, and improves the overall patient billing experience. Here are key considerations for creating clear and transparent patient statements:

1. Use Patient-Friendly Language:

Avoid using complex medical terminology or jargon that may confuse patients. Instead, use plain language that patients can easily understand. Clearly explain services rendered, charges, and any insurance adjustments or denials in simple terms.

2. Itemized Billing:

Provide an itemized breakdown of the services and corresponding charges. Categorize the services by date, type, and cost, enabling patients to review and validate the charges. This breakdown helps patients understand the components of their bill and identify any discrepancies.

3. Include Insurance Payments and Adjustments:

Clearly display any insurance payments or adjustments made on the patient statement. Itemize the insurance payments and indicate the portion covered by insurance and the patient's responsibility. This transparency helps patients understand the financial impact of their insurance coverage.

4. Patient Responsibility:

Clearly outline the patient's financial responsibility, including deductibles, co-pays, co-insurance, or any outstanding balances. Clearly indicate the amount owed by the patient and the due date for payment. This information empowers patients to understand their financial obligations.

5. Explain Codes and Abbreviations:

If there are codes or abbreviations used in the billing statement, provide an explanation key or legend to help patients interpret them. For example, provide a brief description of common procedure codes or abbreviations used for clarity.

6. Payment Options and Instructions:

Clearly state the available payment options, such as online payment portals, credit card payments, checks, or payment plans. Provide step-by-step instructions on how to make payments, including the necessary account details and contact information for assistance.

7. Contact Information:

Include clear contact information, such as phone numbers or email addresses, for patients to reach out with questions or concerns. Provide dedicated customer service or billing department contact details to facilitate timely resolution of billing inquiries.

8. Financial Assistance Programs:

If the healthcare organization offers financial assistance programs or payment assistance options, clearly outline the eligibility criteria and application process. Provide information on how patients can inquire about and apply for financial assistance if needed.

9. Visual Design and Layout:

Design the patient statement with a clean and organized layout. Use headings, subheadings, and bullet points to structure the information clearly. Utilize easy-to-read fonts and appropriate font sizes. Consider using colors or highlighting techniques to draw attention to important sections or payment due dates.

10. Patient Education Materials:

Include supplemental educational materials or resources that explain common billing terms, insurance coverage basics, or frequently asked questions related to the patient statement. Provide patients with access to additional resources or online tools to enhance their understanding of the billing process.

11. Test and Seek Patient Feedback:

Test the clarity and effectiveness of the patient statement with a sample group of patients. Gather feedback on the readability, comprehensibility, and overall satisfaction with the statement format and content. Use this feedback to refine and improve the patient statement design and content.

Creating clear and transparent patient statements promotes patient engagement, reduces billing inquiries, and increases the likelihood of prompt and accurate payments. Regularly assess patient feedback, review industry best practices, and make necessary updates to the patient statement design and content for ongoing improvement.

Patient collections strategies and financial assistance programs play a crucial role in managing outstanding patient balances and facilitating timely payment. By implementing effective collections strategies and offering financial assistance options, healthcare organizations can improve their revenue cycle performance and support patients facing financial challenges. Here are key strategies and considerations:

1. Clear Communication:

Establish clear and transparent communication with patients regarding their financial responsibility. Clearly explain the billing process, payment expectations, and available payment options. Provide patients with a breakdown of charges and assist them in understanding insurance coverage, deductibles, co-pays, and any outstanding balances.

2. Payment Options:

Offer a range of convenient payment options to accommodate patient preferences. Provide multiple channels for payment, such as online portals, credit card payments, electronic fund transfers, checks, or payment plans. Make it easy for patients to make payments and provide clear instructions for each payment option.

3. Financial Counseling:

Provide financial counseling services to help patients navigate their medical bills and explore available options. Trained financial counselors can assist patients in understanding their insurance coverage, eligibility for financial assistance programs, and the process of applying for assistance.

4. Financial Assistance Programs:

Establish financial assistance programs to support patients with limited financial resources. Develop clear guidelines and criteria for eligibility, income-based sliding scales, or charity care programs. Communicate the availability of these programs to patients and provide assistance with the application process.

5. Eligibility Determination:

Implement a systematic process for determining patient eligibility for financial assistance programs. Evaluate patients' financial situations and verify their eligibility based on predetermined criteria. Maintain confidentiality and sensitivity when handling patient financial information.

6. Payment Plans and Negotiation:

Offer flexible payment plans tailored to patients' financial capabilities. Work with patients to establish manageable payment schedules based on their income and expenses. Consider negotiating reduced payment amounts or settlements for patients experiencing financial hardship.

7. Early Intervention:

Implement early intervention strategies to address potential payment issues. Proactively communicate with patients to remind them of their financial obligations, offer assistance, and address any concerns or questions they may have. Identify patients who may need additional support and reach out to them before their balances become delinquent.

8. Collections Policies and Procedures:

Develop clear collections policies and procedures that outline the steps for escalating collections efforts when payment is overdue. Establish guidelines for when and how to engage external collections agencies, if necessary. Ensure compliance with relevant laws and regulations governing collections practices.

9. Staff Training:

Provide training for staff involved in patient collections to ensure they possess the necessary skills and sensitivity to handle financial discussions with patients. Train staff members on effective communication techniques, negotiation strategies, and empathy when addressing patient financial concerns.

10. Compliance with Regulations:

Ensure compliance with federal and state regulations, including the Fair Debt Collection Practices Act (FDCPA) and the Health Insurance Portability and Accountability Act (HIPAA). Protect patient privacy and maintain confidentiality when discussing financial matters.

11. Regular Analysis and Process Improvement:

Continuously analyze collections data and key performance indicators (KPIs) to assess the effectiveness of patient collections strategies. Identify trends, bottlenecks, and areas for improvement. Implement process enhancements based on data analysis to streamline collections and enhance patient satisfaction.

By implementing these patient collections strategies and offering financial assistance programs, healthcare organizations can support patients in managing their medical bills, improve revenue recovery, and maintain positive patient experiences. Regularly review and update collections policies and procedures to align with industry best practices and evolving patient needs.

Exercise 11: Patient Billing and Collections

1. Overview of Patient Billing Cycle

Question 1: What is the purpose of the patient billing cycle in revenue cycle management (RCM)?

Answer: The purpose of the patient billing cycle in RCM is to generate and deliver accurate and timely bills to patients for the healthcare services they have received. The patient billing cycle encompasses various steps, including capturing charges, verifying insurance coverage, determining patient financial responsibility, generating statements, and collecting payments. It aims to ensure that patients are aware of their financial obligations and to facilitate the timely and accurate collection of payments for services rendered.

Question 2: What are the key steps involved in the patient billing cycle?

Answer: The key steps involved in the patient billing cycle include:

- Charge capture: Recording and documenting the services provided to the patient.

- Insurance verification: Verifying the patient's insurance coverage and determining the patient's financial responsibility.

- Claims submission: Submitting claims to insurance payers for reimbursement.

- Adjudication: The process by which insurance payers review and evaluate claims for reimbursement.

- Explanation of Benefits (EOB): Providing patients with a summary of how their claims were processed and any patient responsibility.

- Patient statement generation: Generating clear and detailed statements that outline the patient's financial responsibility.

- Payment collection: Collecting payments from patients through various methods, such as cash, check, credit card, or online payments.

- Follow-up and collections: Following up with patients who have outstanding balances and implementing collections strategies to collect overdue payments.

2. Clear and Transparent Patient Statements

Question 1: Why is it important to provide clear and transparent patient statements in revenue cycle management (RCM)?

Answer: Providing clear and transparent patient statements is important in RCM because:

- It helps patients understand the charges, services provided, and their financial responsibility.

- It promotes transparency and builds trust between patients and healthcare organizations.

- It reduces the risk of billing errors and disputes by clearly presenting the details of the services and charges.

- It improves patient satisfaction by providing easy-to-understand statements that facilitate payment processing.

- It enhances the likelihood of timely payments by minimizing confusion and encouraging prompt resolution of outstanding balances.

- It supports compliance with regulatory requirements, such as providing accurate and itemized statements as mandated by law.

Question 2: What are some best practices for creating clear and transparent patient statements?

Answer: Some best practices for creating clear and transparent patient statements include:

- Using plain language and avoiding complex medical terminology or jargon.

- Presenting charges in an itemized format, clearly indicating the services provided and their associated costs.

- Providing a clear breakdown of insurance coverage, adjustments, and patient responsibility.

- Including payment due dates, accepted payment methods, and instructions for making payments.

- Offering multiple channels for accessing statements, such as print, online portals, or mobile applications.

- Incorporating visual elements, such as charts or graphs, to enhance clarity and understanding.

- Ensuring consistency in the layout and design of statements to facilitate ease of reading and comprehension.

- Including contact information for billing inquiries or assistance to address patient concerns promptly.

3. Patient Collections Strategies and Financial Assistance

Question 1: What are some patient collections strategies that can be implemented to improve revenue collection in healthcare?

Answer: Some patient collections strategies that can be implemented to improve revenue collection in healthcare include:

- Establishing clear payment policies and communicating them to patients upfront.

- Offering convenient payment options, such as online payment portals, automated payment plans, or credit card on file programs.

- Implementing financial counseling and education programs to help patients understand their financial responsibilities and explore available payment options.

- Utilizing patient engagement tools, such as appointment reminders or patient portals, to proactively communicate about outstanding balances and payment due dates.

- Implementing a structured collections process, including reminders, phone calls, or collection letters, for patients with unpaid balances.

- Collaborating with patient advocacy organizations or financial assistance programs to identify resources for patients who are unable to pay.

- Training staff on effective communication and customer service skills to handle sensitive financial discussions with patients.

- Offering flexible payment arrangements or financial hardship programs for patients facing financial difficulties.

Question 2: What is the significance of providing financial assistance programs in revenue cycle management (RCM)?

Answer: Providing financial assistance programs in RCM is significant because:

- It ensures that patients with financial constraints can access necessary healthcare services without undue financial burden.

- It supports the organization's commitment to providing equitable and accessible care for all patients, regardless of their financial status.

- It helps reduce the likelihood of bad debt write-offs and uncollectible accounts by offering alternative payment options or forgiveness programs.

- It fosters positive patient experiences and satisfaction by demonstrating compassion and understanding toward patients' financial circumstances.

- It contributes to the organization's reputation and community goodwill by being socially responsible and responsive to the needs of underserved populations.

- It aligns with regulatory requirements and guidelines, such as providing financial assistance to eligible patients as mandated by law.

These exercises provide an opportunity to reinforce the knowledge gained from the chapter on Patient Billing and Collections. The questions assess understanding and reinforce key concepts related to the overview of the patient billing cycle, creating clear and transparent patient statements, and implementing patient collections strategies and financial assistance programs in revenue cycle management.

12. Financial Assistance and Charity Care

12.1 Overview of Financial Assistance Programs:

Financial assistance programs, including charity care, are designed to support individuals who are unable to pay for their medical services due to financial hardship. These programs help ensure that patients have access to necessary healthcare services regardless of their ability to pay. Here's an overview of financial assistance programs:

1. Definition and Purpose:

Financial assistance programs provide reduced-cost or free healthcare services to individuals who meet specific eligibility criteria based on their financial circumstances. The primary purpose is to assist individuals facing financial hardship and ensure they receive necessary medical care without incurring overwhelming financial burdens.

2. Eligibility Criteria:

Financial assistance programs typically have specific eligibility criteria that consider factors such as income, household size, and assets. These criteria vary among healthcare organizations and are designed to determine the level of financial need. Eligibility is assessed through an application process and often requires supporting documentation, such as income tax returns or pay stubs.

3. Sliding Fee Scales:

Many financial assistance programs utilize sliding fee scales to determine the level of assistance based on the patient's income. The sliding fee scale takes into account the patient's income level and assigns a corresponding discount percentage, which reduces the patient's financial responsibility for healthcare services.

4. Charity Care:

Charity care refers to the provision of free or significantly reduced-cost healthcare services to individuals who meet the eligibility criteria of a healthcare organization's charitable care policy. Charity care programs are typically reserved for patients with the most significant financial need and are funded through the healthcare organization's charitable contributions or budget allocations.

5. Application Process:

Healthcare organizations establish an application process for patients seeking financial assistance. This process typically involves completing an application form, submitting supporting documentation, and providing proof of financial need. The application is reviewed by the healthcare organization's financial assistance department or designated personnel.

6. Confidentiality:

Maintaining patient confidentiality is a crucial aspect of financial assistance programs. Patient information, including financial and medical records, should be handled with strict confidentiality and in compliance with applicable privacy laws and regulations, such as HIPAA.

7. Communication and Patient Education:

Effective communication is vital in ensuring patients are aware of the availability of financial assistance programs. Healthcare organizations should clearly communicate the existence, eligibility criteria, application process, and benefits of the program. Patient education materials, including brochures or online resources, can help individuals understand their options and guide them through the application process.

8. Community Partnerships:

Healthcare organizations often collaborate with community organizations, nonprofits, and government agencies to expand the reach of financial assistance programs. These partnerships help identify individuals in need, provide referrals, and ensure a coordinated approach to addressing community health needs.

9. Compliance and Reporting:

Healthcare organizations must comply with applicable laws and regulations governing financial assistance programs. This includes transparency in financial reporting, adhering to tax-exempt status requirements, and maintaining appropriate documentation to demonstrate compliance with charity care obligations.

10. Ongoing Evaluation and Improvement:

Financial assistance programs should undergo regular evaluation to assess their effectiveness and make necessary improvements. This includes monitoring patient satisfaction, reviewing program outcomes, and incorporating feedback from applicants and staff to enhance program efficiency and accessibility.

Financial assistance programs and charity care play a crucial role in promoting equitable access to healthcare services for individuals experiencing financial hardship. By implementing well-designed programs, healthcare organizations can alleviate the financial burden on patients, improve community health outcomes, and fulfill their mission of providing compassionate care to all individuals in need.

12.2 Eligibility Criteria and Application Process:

Eligibility criteria and the application process are key components of financial assistance programs. They determine who qualifies for assistance based on their financial circumstances and guide the application process. Here's an overview of eligibility criteria and the application process for financial assistance programs:

Eligibility Criteria:

1. Income Level:

Financial assistance programs typically consider the applicant's income level as a primary factor in determining eligibility. Income limits are set based on federal poverty guidelines or specific income thresholds established by the healthcare organization. The income limits may vary depending on family size and household income.

2. Assets and Resources:

Some programs may consider the applicant's assets and resources in addition to income. This can include savings accounts, investments, property ownership, or other financial resources. The specific asset limits or exclusions are defined by the healthcare organization and may vary.

3. Insurance Coverage:

Financial assistance programs often take into account whether the applicant has health insurance coverage. They may target individuals who are uninsured, have limited insurance coverage, or face high out-of-pocket expenses. The program may also consider the availability of Medicaid or other government assistance programs.

4. Residency and Citizenship:

Eligibility may require proof of residency within a defined geographic area served by the healthcare organization. In some cases, citizenship or immigration status may also be considered. Non-discrimination policies ensure that individuals are not excluded based on their immigration status.

5. Medical Necessity:

Financial assistance programs typically focus on covering services that are medically necessary. The program may consider whether the services rendered align with accepted medical guidelines and are appropriate for the patient's condition.

Application Process:

1. Application Form:

Applicants must complete an application form provided by the healthcare organization. The form collects information about the applicant's household size, income, assets, insurance coverage, and other relevant details. It may also require supporting documentation, such as pay stubs, tax returns, or bank statements.

2. Supporting Documentation:

Applicants are typically required to submit supporting documentation to verify their income and financial circumstances. The specific documentation required may vary but can include recent tax returns, W-2 forms, bank statements, or other proof of income and assets. Clear instructions on the required documentation should be provided to applicants.

3. Application Submission:

The completed application form and supporting documentation are submitted to the healthcare organization's financial assistance department or designated personnel. The submission process may involve mailing the application, submitting it in person, or utilizing an online application portal, if available.

4. Application Review:

The healthcare organization's financial assistance department reviews the application and supporting documentation. They assess the applicant's financial need based on the eligibility criteria defined by the program. The review process may involve verifying income, assets, insurance coverage, and any other relevant information.

5. Notification of Eligibility:

After reviewing the application, the healthcare organization notifies the applicant of their eligibility status. This can be done through written communication, phone calls, or electronic notifications. If eligible, the notification will include details of the financial assistance benefits offered.

6. Appeals Process:

In the case of an application denial, healthcare organizations typically have an appeals process in place. Applicants can request a reconsideration of their eligibility determination by providing additional information or addressing any discrepancies that may have impacted the initial decision.

7. Confidentiality:

Confidentiality of applicant information is crucial during the application process. Healthcare organizations should have safeguards in place to protect the privacy of applicants, adhere to HIPAA regulations, and ensure that only authorized personnel have access to sensitive information.

8. Patient Assistance and Guidance:

Throughout the application process, healthcare organizations should provide assistance and guidance to applicants. This can include offering resources, explaining the application requirements, answering questions, and providing support to ensure applicants understand and complete the process successfully.

Clear communication of eligibility criteria, a well-defined application process, and compassionate support are essential in making financial assistance programs accessible to those in need. Healthcare organizations should continuously evaluate and improve their application processes to streamline workflows, enhance efficiency, and provide a positive experience for applicants seeking financial assistance.

12.3 Compliance with Regulatory Requirements:

Compliance with regulatory requirements is crucial for financial assistance programs to ensure fair and equitable access to healthcare services and to maintain the organization's tax-exempt status. Healthcare organizations offering financial assistance programs must adhere to various laws, regulations, and guidelines. Here are key considerations for compliance:

1. Internal Revenue Service (IRS) Regulations:

Healthcare organizations must comply with IRS regulations to maintain their tax-exempt status and qualify for certain tax benefits. This includes adherence to the community benefit standard, which requires providing a significant level of uncompensated care and offering financial assistance programs to individuals who meet the organization's eligibility criteria.

2. Patient Protection and Affordable Care Act (ACA):

The ACA includes provisions related to financial assistance programs, such as the requirement to establish a written financial assistance policy and limit charges to individuals eligible for financial assistance. Healthcare organizations must comply with these provisions to ensure compliance with the law.

3. State and Local Regulations:

Healthcare organizations should be familiar with state and local regulations governing financial assistance programs. These regulations may vary across jurisdictions and may include requirements related to eligibility criteria, program administration, disclosure requirements, and compliance with consumer protection laws.

4. Anti-Discrimination Laws:

Financial assistance programs must comply with federal and state anti-discrimination laws, such as the Civil Rights Act of 1964 and the Americans with Disabilities Act (ADA). Eligibility criteria, application processes, and program administration must not discriminate against individuals based on factors such as race, color, national origin, disability, or religion.

5. Health Insurance Portability and Accountability Act (HIPAA):

Compliance with HIPAA regulations is critical in protecting the privacy and security of patient information. Healthcare organizations must ensure that all patient information collected during the financial assistance application process is handled in accordance with HIPAA requirements. Safeguards should be in place to protect the confidentiality of applicant information.

6. Fair Debt Collection Practices Act (FDCPA):

Healthcare organizations engaging in collection activities related to outstanding patient balances must comply with the FDCPA. This federal law regulates the conduct of debt collectors and sets standards for fair and ethical debt collection practices, including limitations on harassment, misrepresentation, and unfair collection methods.

7. Transparency and Disclosure Requirements:

Financial assistance programs must provide clear and transparent information to patients regarding the availability, eligibility criteria, application process, and benefits of the program. Organizations should ensure that program information is readily accessible and easily understandable to patients, promoting transparency and informed decision-making.

8. Compliance Reporting and Documentation:

Healthcare organizations offering financial assistance programs should maintain comprehensive documentation and records to demonstrate compliance with regulatory requirements. This includes documenting policies, procedures, eligibility determinations, application reviews, and any other relevant information. Regular reporting may be required to demonstrate compliance with community benefit obligations.

9. Regular Audits and Internal Controls:

Conducting regular audits and implementing internal controls are essential to ensure ongoing compliance with regulatory requirements. Audits help identify any gaps or areas for improvement, while internal controls help maintain consistency, accuracy, and integrity in program administration.

10. Staff Training and Education:

Ensure that staff members involved in financial assistance program administration receive appropriate training and education on regulatory requirements, including compliance, patient privacy, and fair debt collection practices. Ongoing training helps promote compliance awareness and ensures consistent adherence to regulatory guidelines.

Compliance with regulatory requirements is crucial to protect the integrity of financial assistance programs and maintain the trust of patients and the community. Healthcare organizations should regularly review and update their policies and procedures to align with evolving regulations and industry best practices.

Exercise 12: Financial Assistance and Charity Care

1. Overview of Financial Assistance Programs

Question 1: What is the purpose of financial assistance programs in revenue cycle management (RCM)?

Answer: The purpose of financial assistance programs in RCM is to provide support and financial relief to patients who are unable to afford the full cost of healthcare services. These programs aim to ensure access to necessary care for individuals who face financial hardships, promoting equitable healthcare delivery. Financial assistance programs may involve discounts, reduced payment plans, or charity care options for eligible patients.

Question 2: What are some key benefits of implementing financial assistance programs in healthcare organizations?

Answer: Some key benefits of implementing financial assistance programs in healthcare organizations include:

- Ensuring access to healthcare services for patients who cannot afford to pay the full cost of care.

- Demonstrating social responsibility and commitment to community well-being.

- Enhancing patient satisfaction and loyalty by addressing financial barriers to care.

- Minimizing the risk of bad debt write-offs and uncollectible accounts.

- Complying with regulatory requirements and guidelines related to providing financial assistance to eligible patients.

- Building positive community relationships and fostering goodwill.

2. Eligibility Criteria and Application Process

Question 1: What are some common eligibility criteria for financial assistance programs in healthcare organizations?

Answer: Common eligibility criteria for financial assistance programs in healthcare organizations may include:

- Demonstrated financial need, typically based on income level or household size.

- Lack of insurance coverage or inadequate coverage for specific services.

- Ineligibility for government-funded healthcare programs, such as Medicaid or Medicare.

- Citizenship or residency requirements, depending on the organization's policies.

- Compliance with the organization's application process and documentation requirements.

Question 2: What is the general application process for patients seeking financial assistance?

Answer: The general application process for patients seeking financial assistance may include the following steps:

- Patient inquiry: Patients express their interest in financial assistance and request information or an application form.

- Application submission: Patients complete the financial assistance application form, providing the required documentation and information.

- Documentation review: The healthcare organization reviews the application and supporting documents to determine the patient's eligibility.

- Decision and notification: The organization assesses the application and notifies the patient of the decision regarding their eligibility for financial assistance.

- Communication of benefits: If eligible, the organization communicates the financial assistance benefits to the patient, including any discounts, reduced payment plans, or charity care options.

- Agreement and enrollment: The patient and the organization may enter into an agreement or enrollment process, outlining the terms and conditions of the financial assistance program.

3. Compliance with Regulatory Requirements

Question 1: What are some regulatory requirements and guidelines related to financial assistance programs in healthcare organizations?

Answer: Some regulatory requirements and guidelines related to financial assistance programs in healthcare organizations may include:

- Compliance with federal and state laws regarding charity care and financial assistance, such as the Internal Revenue Service (IRS) guidelines for nonprofit organizations.

- Compliance with regulations related to patient billing and collections, such as the Fair Debt Collection Practices Act (FDCPA) and the Health Insurance Portability and Accountability Act (HIPAA).

- Implementation of policies and procedures to ensure consistent application of financial assistance guidelines and criteria.

- Documentation and reporting requirements to demonstrate compliance with regulatory guidelines.

- Regular audits and reviews to assess the effectiveness and compliance of financial assistance programs.

Question 2: Why is compliance with regulatory requirements important for financial assistance programs in healthcare organizations?

Answer: Compliance with regulatory requirements is important for financial assistance programs in healthcare organizations because:

- It ensures adherence to legal and ethical standards in providing financial assistance to eligible patients.

- It helps organizations maintain their tax-exempt status and comply with reporting requirements for nonprofit entities.

- It protects patients' rights and privacy by complying with regulations related to billing, collections, and patient information confidentiality.

- It minimizes the risk of legal and financial repercussions, such as penalties or lawsuits, resulting from non-compliance.

- It promotes transparency and accountability in financial assistance programs, enhancing public trust and confidence in the organization's operations.

These exercises provide an opportunity to reinforce the knowledge gained from the chapter on Financial Assistance and Charity Care. The questions assess understanding and reinforce key concepts related to the overview of financial assistance programs, eligibility criteria and application processes, and compliance with regulatory requirements in revenue cycle management.

13. Healthcare Compliance and Regulatory Considerations

13.1 HIPAA and Patient Data Privacy:

HIPAA (Health Insurance Portability and Accountability Act) is a federal law enacted in 1996 to protect the privacy and security of patients' health information. Compliance with HIPAA regulations is essential for healthcare organizations to ensure the confidentiality, integrity, and availability of patient data. Here's an overview of HIPAA and its impact on patient data privacy:

1. Protected Health Information (PHI):

HIPAA defines Protected Health Information (PHI) as individually identifiable health information transmitted or maintained by a covered entity or its business associates. PHI includes demographic data, medical records, lab results, insurance information, and other personally identifiable health information.

2. Privacy Rule:

HIPAA Privacy Rule establishes standards for protecting patients' PHI. It grants individuals certain rights regarding their health information and restricts the use and disclosure of PHI by covered entities. The Privacy Rule requires healthcare organizations to implement safeguards to protect the privacy of PHI.

3. Security Rule:

HIPAA Security Rule complements the Privacy Rule and establishes standards for safeguarding electronic PHI (ePHI). It requires healthcare organizations to implement administrative, physical, and technical safeguards to ensure the confidentiality, integrity, and availability of ePHI. This includes measures such as access controls, encryption, and regular risk assessments.

4. Privacy Notice:

Healthcare organizations must provide patients with a Privacy Notice, also known as a Notice of Privacy Practices. This notice explains how their health information will be used, disclosed, and protected. It outlines patients' rights, including the right to access their health information and request amendments or restrictions.

5. Business Associate Agreements:

Covered entities must have Business Associate Agreements (BAAs) in place with vendors or business associates that handle PHI on their behalf. These agreements ensure that business associates comply with HIPAA requirements and adequately protect PHI.

6. Patient Consent:

HIPAA requires patient consent for certain uses and disclosures of PHI. Covered entities must obtain written authorization from patients before using or disclosing their PHI for purposes not covered under the Privacy Rule's exceptions. Patients have the right to revoke their authorization at any time.

7. Breach Notification:

HIPAA mandates that covered entities notify affected individuals, the Department of Health and Human Services (HHS), and potentially the media in the event of a breach of unsecured PHI. Breach notification requirements specify the timeline and content of breach notifications.

8. Enforcement and Penalties:

HHS Office for Civil Rights (OCR) is responsible for enforcing HIPAA compliance. Non-compliance with HIPAA can result in significant penalties, ranging from monetary fines to criminal charges, depending on the severity of the violation.

9. Staff Training:

Healthcare organizations must provide comprehensive training to their workforce on HIPAA regulations, including patient privacy, security awareness, and handling of PHI. Training ensures staff members understand their responsibilities and obligations under HIPAA and helps prevent accidental breaches or non-compliance.

10. Technology and Security Measures:

Healthcare organizations should implement robust technology and security measures to protect PHI. This includes using secure electronic health record (EHR) systems, implementing strong access controls, employing encryption and firewalls, conducting regular security assessments, and implementing policies for secure disposal of PHI.

Compliance with HIPAA regulations is critical to protect patient privacy and maintain the trust of individuals seeking healthcare services. Healthcare organizations should establish comprehensive HIPAA compliance programs, conduct regular audits, and stay updated on any changes or updates to HIPAA regulations to ensure ongoing compliance and patient data privacy.

Healthcare organizations and providers are subject to various anti-fraud and abuse regulations that aim to prevent fraudulent activities and ensure the integrity of healthcare services. Two important regulations in this regard are the Stark Law and the False Claims Act. Here's an overview of these regulations and their impact on healthcare compliance:

1. Stark Law (Physician Self-Referral Law):

The Stark Law prohibits physicians from referring Medicare or Medicaid patients to entities for designated health services (DHS) in which they have a financial interest. It also prohibits entities from submitting claims for services arising from such prohibited referrals. Key aspects of the Stark Law include:

a. Prohibition on Self-Referrals: Physicians are prohibited from referring Medicare or Medicaid patients for certain designated health services to entities with which they have a financial relationship, unless an exception applies.

b. Financial Relationships: Financial relationships subject to the Stark Law include ownership or investment interests, compensation arrangements, and certain exceptions for employment relationships and personal services arrangements.

c. Strict Liability: Violations of the Stark Law are considered strict liability offenses, meaning intent or knowledge of the violation is not required for penalties to be imposed.

Compliance with the Stark Law is crucial to avoid potential penalties, including exclusion from Medicare and Medicaid programs, recoupment of payments, and civil monetary penalties.

2. False Claims Act (FCA):

The False Claims Act is a federal law that imposes liability on individuals and entities that submit false or fraudulent claims for payment to the government. It prohibits the knowing submission of false claims and imposes significant penalties for violations. Key aspects of the False Claims Act include:

a. Prohibition on False Claims: It is illegal to knowingly submit false or fraudulent claims to government healthcare programs, such as Medicare and Medicaid. This includes claims for services not provided, claims with false information, or claims that violate other regulations.

b. Whistleblower Provisions: The False Claims Act allows private individuals, known as whistleblowers or relators, to file lawsuits on behalf of the government to recover funds lost due to false claims. Whistleblowers may receive a portion of the recovered funds as a reward.

c. Penalties and Liability: Violations of the False Claims Act can result in substantial penalties, including treble damages (three times the amount of damages suffered by the government), fines, and potential exclusion from government healthcare programs.

Compliance with the False Claims Act requires healthcare organizations to establish effective compliance programs, conduct regular audits and monitoring, and ensure accurate and truthful billing practices.

3. Anti-Kickback Statute:

The Anti-Kickback Statute prohibits offering, paying, soliciting, or receiving remuneration in exchange for referrals or generating business reimbursed by federal healthcare programs. The statute is aimed at preventing illegal kickback arrangements that could influence medical decision-making and lead to overutilization or improper billing.

Compliance with the Anti-Kickback Statute is essential for healthcare organizations to avoid penalties, including criminal and civil liability, fines, and exclusion from government healthcare programs.

4. Compliance Programs and Audits:

To ensure compliance with anti-fraud and abuse regulations, healthcare organizations should establish robust compliance programs that include policies, procedures, and training to prevent, detect, and respond to potential violations. Regular audits and monitoring can help identify and address any potential compliance issues.

5. Reporting and Investigation:

Healthcare organizations should have mechanisms in place to encourage the reporting of suspected fraudulent activities internally and to appropriate regulatory authorities. Prompt investigation and appropriate action in response to suspected violations are essential to demonstrate a commitment to compliance.

Compliance with anti-fraud and abuse regulations, including the Stark Law and the False Claims Act, is crucial to maintain the integrity of healthcare services and avoid legal and financial repercussions. Healthcare organizations should stay informed about these regulations, establish comprehensive compliance programs, and seek legal counsel when necessary to ensure ongoing compliance with the law.

13.3 RCM Compliance Audits and Monitoring:

Compliance audits and monitoring are essential components of an effective revenue cycle management (RCM) program. They help ensure that healthcare organizations adhere to regulatory requirements, internal policies, and industry best practices. Here's an overview of RCM compliance audits and monitoring:

1. Purpose of Compliance Audits and Monitoring:

Compliance audits and monitoring activities aim to assess the effectiveness of RCM processes, identify areas of non-compliance, mitigate financial and legal risks, and promote a culture of compliance within the organization. These activities help ensure that RCM practices align with applicable laws, regulations, and internal policies.

2. Establishing a Compliance Audit Plan:

Healthcare organizations should develop a comprehensive compliance audit plan specific to RCM. The plan should outline the scope, objectives, frequency, and methodology of the audits. It should consider key areas such as billing and coding accuracy, documentation completeness, claim submission and reimbursement, contractual compliance, and adherence to regulatory requirements.

3. Conducting Compliance Audits:

Compliance audits involve a systematic review of RCM processes, documentation, and related activities. Audits can be conducted internally by a dedicated compliance team or externally by independent auditors. The audits should follow established protocols and include a combination of random and targeted sampling to assess compliance.

4. Compliance Monitoring:

Compliance monitoring involves ongoing surveillance of RCM processes to identify and address compliance issues in real-time. This can be achieved through continuous monitoring tools, data analytics, and regular assessments of key performance indicators (KPIs). Monitoring activities should focus on critical areas such as coding accuracy, claim submission, reimbursement trends, and denials management.

5. Documentation Review:

Compliance audits and monitoring involve reviewing documentation related to RCM processes, including patient records, coding and billing records, claims, reimbursement documentation, and contracts with payers. The review assesses the accuracy, completeness, and compliance with relevant regulations and internal policies.

6. Internal Controls and Policies:

Compliance audits and monitoring evaluate the effectiveness of internal controls and policies related to RCM. This includes assessing the design and implementation of controls to prevent and detect non-compliance, such as segregation of duties, documentation standards, authorization processes, and oversight mechanisms.

7. External Regulatory Compliance:

Compliance audits and monitoring should ensure adherence to external regulatory requirements, such as HIPAA, Stark Law, False Claims Act, and other relevant regulations specific to RCM. The audits assess the organization's compliance with these regulations, including patient data privacy, self-referral prohibitions, accurate claims submission, and fraud prevention.

8. Remediation and Corrective Actions:

Compliance audits and monitoring activities should result in the identification of non-compliance issues. In such cases, appropriate remediation and corrective actions should be implemented promptly. This may involve updating policies and procedures, providing additional training, enhancing internal controls, or addressing gaps in processes.

9. Training and Education:

Compliance audits and monitoring help identify areas where staff members may require additional training and education. This enables organizations to provide targeted training programs to improve understanding and compliance with RCM processes and regulatory requirements.

10. Reporting and Follow-up:

Compliance audit findings and monitoring results should be documented and reported to the appropriate stakeholders, such as senior management, compliance officers, and relevant departments. The organization should establish a follow-up process to ensure timely resolution of identified issues and track the implementation of remedial actions.

11. Continuous Improvement:

Compliance audits and monitoring activities should be viewed as ongoing processes. Regularly reviewing audit findings, monitoring results, and incorporating lessons learned into RCM processes allows for continuous improvement of compliance efforts.

Compliance audits and monitoring provide valuable insights into the effectiveness of RCM processes, identify areas for improvement, and help ensure adherence to regulatory requirements. By conducting regular audits, implementing monitoring mechanisms, and taking corrective actions, healthcare organizations can strengthen their compliance efforts and minimize risks in the revenue cycle management process.

Exercise 13: Healthcare Compliance and Regulatory Considerations

1. HIPAA and Patient Data Privacy

Question 1: What does HIPAA stand for, and what is its significance in healthcare compliance?

Answer: HIPAA stands for the Health Insurance Portability and Accountability Act. It is a federal law in the United States that sets standards and regulations for protecting the privacy and security of patients' health information. HIPAA's significance in healthcare compliance includes:

- Safeguarding patients' sensitive health information from unauthorized access, use, or disclosure.

- Promoting patients' rights and control over their health information.

- Establishing rules for healthcare organizations and providers to ensure the confidentiality, integrity, and availability of patient data.

- Requiring healthcare organizations to implement administrative, physical, and technical safeguards to protect patient information.

- Mandating the use of secure electronic transactions and privacy practices in healthcare operations.

Question 2: What are some key provisions of HIPAA related to patient data privacy?

Answer: Some key provisions of HIPAA related to patient data privacy include:

- Privacy Rule: The Privacy Rule sets standards for the protection of individually identifiable health information, including the rights of patients to access their records, control the use and disclosure of their information, and be informed of their privacy rights.

- Security Rule: The Security Rule establishes standards for the security of electronic protected health information (ePHI) and requires the implementation of safeguards to protect against unauthorized access, use, or disclosure.

- Breach Notification Rule: The Breach Notification Rule requires covered entities to notify affected individuals, the Secretary of Health and Human Services, and, in some cases, the media in the event of a breach of unsecured protected health information.

- Enforcement: HIPAA provides for civil and criminal penalties for non-compliance, including fines and imprisonment, to ensure adherence to the regulations.

2. Anti-Fraud and Abuse Regulations (e.g., Stark Law, False Claims Act)

Question 1: What is the Stark Law, and how does it relate to healthcare compliance?

Answer: The Stark Law, also known as the Physician Self-Referral Law, is a federal law in the United States that prohibits physicians from referring Medicare patients for certain designated health services to entities with which they have financial relationships, unless specific exceptions apply. The Stark Law aims to prevent self-referral arrangements that may lead to inappropriate utilization and increased healthcare costs. Compliance with the Stark Law is crucial in healthcare to ensure adherence to anti-fraud and abuse regulations and to avoid penalties for non-compliance.

Question 2: What is the False Claims Act, and why is it significant in healthcare compliance?

Answer: The False Claims Act is a federal law that imposes liability on individuals or organizations that submit false or fraudulent claims for payment to the government, including Medicare or Medicaid. The False Claims Act is significant in healthcare compliance because it encourages the detection and prevention of fraud and abuse in healthcare programs. Violations of the False Claims Act can result in significant penalties, including monetary fines and exclusion from participation in government healthcare programs.

3. RCM Compliance Audits and Monitoring

Question 1: What is the purpose of RCM compliance audits in healthcare organizations?

Answer: The purpose of RCM compliance audits in healthcare organizations is to assess the organization's adherence to applicable laws, regulations, and internal policies related to revenue cycle management. Compliance audits help identify areas of non-compliance, vulnerabilities, or weaknesses in processes and controls, allowing organizations to take corrective actions and mitigate compliance risks. Audits also serve as a proactive measure to monitor and ensure compliance with regulatory requirements, maintain the integrity of financial operations, and safeguard against fraud and abuse.

Question 2: What are some key elements of RCM compliance monitoring programs?

Answer: Key elements of RCM compliance monitoring programs include:

- Regular monitoring and analysis of revenue cycle processes and transactions to identify potential compliance issues.

- Utilization of data analytics and software tools to identify patterns or anomalies that may indicate non-compliance.

- Conducting internal audits to assess adherence to regulatory requirements, policies, and industry best practices.

- Implementing effective controls, policies, and procedures to ensure compliance with applicable laws and regulations.

- Staff education and training on compliance requirements and expectations.

- Collaboration with legal and compliance professionals to interpret and address complex regulatory issues.

- Timely and appropriate response to identified compliance issues, including corrective actions and process improvements.

- Documentation and record-keeping of compliance activities and outcomes for reporting and future reference.

These exercises provide an opportunity to reinforce the knowledge gained from the chapter on Healthcare Compliance and Regulatory Considerations. The questions assess understanding and reinforce key concepts related to HIPAA and patient data privacy, anti-fraud and abuse regulations, such as the Stark Law and False Claims Act, and RCM compliance audits and monitoring in revenue cycle management.

14. Technology and Automation in RCM

14.1 RCM Software and Systems Overview:

Technology and automation play a crucial role in optimizing revenue cycle management (RCM) processes. RCM software and systems streamline operations, improve efficiency, enhance accuracy, and provide valuable insights into financial performance. Here's an overview of RCM software and systems commonly used in healthcare organizations:

1. Practice Management Systems (PMS):

Practice Management Systems are comprehensive software solutions designed to manage various aspects of healthcare practice operations, including scheduling, patient registration, billing, and claims management. PMSs integrate multiple functions into a single platform, facilitating seamless coordination and workflow efficiency.

2. Electronic Health Record (EHR) Systems:

EHR systems digitally store and manage patient health records, including medical history, diagnoses, treatment plans, and test results. Integration between EHR and RCM systems enables accurate coding, claims generation, and streamlined revenue cycle workflows.

3. Medical Coding and Documentation Tools:

Medical coding and documentation tools assist healthcare providers in accurately coding procedures, diagnoses, and services. These tools automate the coding process, reducing errors and ensuring compliance with coding guidelines, such as Current Procedural Terminology (CPT), International Classification of Diseases (ICD), and Healthcare Common Procedure Coding System (HCPCS).

4. Claims Management Systems:

Claims management systems streamline the process of submitting, tracking, and managing insurance claims. These systems automate claim generation, validate coding accuracy, and facilitate electronic claim submission to payers. They also provide functionalities for claim status tracking, denial management, and resubmission if necessary.

5. Revenue Cycle Analytics and Reporting Tools:

Revenue cycle analytics and reporting tools provide real-time insights into financial performance, key performance indicators (KPIs), and revenue cycle metrics. These tools enable healthcare organizations to monitor cash flow, identify trends, measure productivity, and make data-driven decisions to improve revenue cycle outcomes.

6. Electronic Remittance Advice (ERA) and Payment Posting Systems:

ERA and payment posting systems automate the process of reconciling payments received from payers with submitted claims. These systems match payment information with the corresponding claims, identify discrepancies, and streamline the payment posting process. They also generate reports and provide detailed payment reconciliation information.

7. Patient Payment Solutions:

Patient payment solutions enable electronic payment processing and facilitate patient financial transactions. These solutions include online payment portals, secure payment gateways, and point-of-service payment systems. They enhance patient convenience, improve payment collection rates, and streamline the revenue cycle for patient payments.

8. Denial Management Systems:

Denial management systems help healthcare organizations identify, track, and manage claim denials. These systems analyze denial patterns, identify root causes, and enable proactive intervention to minimize denials. They provide workflow tools for denial resolution, appeals management, and reporting on denial-related KPIs.

9. Artificial Intelligence (AI) and Machine Learning (ML) Applications:

AI and ML applications are increasingly being integrated into RCM systems to enhance automation, decision support, and predictive analytics. These technologies assist in identifying coding errors, optimizing revenue capture, predicting reimbursement outcomes, and streamlining claims processing.

10. Interoperability and Integration Capabilities:

RCM software and systems should have robust interoperability and integration capabilities to facilitate seamless data exchange with other systems such as EHRs, billing systems, and payer portals. This ensures smooth information flow, reduces manual data entry, and minimizes data errors.

Implementing RCM software and systems streamlines revenue cycle processes, improves accuracy, reduces manual effort, and enhances overall efficiency. However, healthcare organizations should carefully select software solutions that align with their specific needs, consider scalability, and ensure compatibility with existing systems. Regular updates, user training, and ongoing support are also important to maximize the benefits of RCM technology and automation.

14.2 Electronic Health Records (EHR) and Integration:

Electronic Health Records (EHR) are digital versions of patients' medical records that provide comprehensive and accessible information about their health history, diagnoses, treatments, and other relevant data. Integration of EHR systems with revenue cycle management (RCM) processes is essential for efficient and accurate billing, coding, and claims management. Here's an overview of EHR integration in RCM:

1. Data Exchange and Interoperability:

EHR integration involves seamless data exchange and interoperability between the EHR system and RCM software or systems. It allows for the secure transfer of patient data, such as demographics, diagnoses, procedures, and medication information, between the EHR and RCM systems.

2. Patient Registration and Eligibility Verification:

Integration enables the automatic retrieval of patient demographic data from the EHR system during the registration process. This minimizes manual data entry, reduces errors, and improves the accuracy of patient information. Integration also facilitates real-time eligibility verification by connecting with payer systems to confirm insurance coverage and benefits.

3. Accurate Coding and Documentation:

Integration between EHR and coding systems ensures that coding is based on accurate and complete clinical documentation. Relevant information, such as diagnoses, procedures, and medical history, can be automatically extracted from the EHR, supporting accurate code assignment and minimizing coding errors.

4. Claim Generation and Submission:

EHR integration with claims management systems enables the seamless generation and submission of claims based on coded clinical data. This integration streamlines the claims process, reduces manual effort, and improves claim accuracy. Claims can be automatically generated with the required coding and patient information, accelerating the submission process.

5. Real-Time Claim Status and Denial Management:

Integrated systems allow for real-time access to claim status information. When claims are submitted, updates on claim status, including acceptance, processing, or denial, can be obtained directly from payer systems. This facilitates proactive denial management, enabling timely resubmissions or appeals, if necessary.

6. Revenue Capture and Charge Capture:

Integration supports accurate revenue capture by capturing charges directly from the EHR system based on documented services and procedures. This eliminates the need for manual charge entry, reduces errors, and ensures accurate billing based on the provided services.

7. Payment Posting and Reconciliation:

Integrated systems automate payment posting and reconciliation by connecting EHR data with payment and remittance advice (ERA) systems. Payments received from payers can be matched with corresponding claims, and discrepancies can be identified and resolved efficiently. This streamlines the payment reconciliation process and minimizes errors.

8. Documentation Integrity and Compliance:

Integration helps ensure documentation integrity by linking clinical information in the EHR to the corresponding billing and coding data. This promotes accurate and complete documentation, supports compliance with coding guidelines, and minimizes the risk of audits and claims denials due to insufficient documentation.

9. Reporting and Analytics:

Integrated EHR and RCM systems provide enhanced reporting and analytics capabilities. Data from both systems can be combined to generate meaningful insights into financial performance, patient demographics, reimbursement trends, and other key metrics. This empowers healthcare organizations to make data-driven decisions and optimize revenue cycle processes.

10. Streamlined Workflows and Efficiency:

EHR integration streamlines workflows by eliminating redundant data entry and manual handoffs between systems. It reduces administrative burden, improves operational efficiency, and enables staff to focus on patient care rather than administrative tasks.

Successful EHR integration requires careful planning, coordination, and collaboration between IT teams, clinical staff, and revenue cycle management personnel. Regular system updates, data integrity checks, and training are essential to ensure seamless integration and optimize the benefits of EHR integration in revenue cycle management.

14.3 Benefits and Challenges of RCM Automation:

RCM automation, enabled through technology and software solutions, offers numerous benefits for healthcare organizations in streamlining revenue cycle management processes. However, it also presents certain challenges that need to be addressed for successful implementation. Here are the benefits and challenges of RCM automation:

Benefits of RCM Automation:

1. Increased Efficiency and Productivity:

   Automation reduces manual tasks, minimizes paper-based processes, and streamlines workflows, leading to increased operational efficiency and productivity. Staff members can focus on value-added activities rather than repetitive administrative tasks.

2. Improved Accuracy and Reduced Errors:

   Automation reduces the risk of human errors that can occur during manual data entry, coding, and claims submission. It enhances accuracy in billing, coding, and claims management, resulting in fewer denials and improved revenue capture.

3. Faster Claims Processing and Reimbursement:

   Automated systems expedite the claims submission process, enabling faster claim processing by payers. This leads to quicker reimbursement and improved cash flow for healthcare organizations.

4. Enhanced Coding and Documentation Compliance:

   RCM automation systems provide built-in coding and documentation compliance checks, ensuring adherence to coding guidelines, regulatory requirements, and payer policies. This reduces the risk of compliance-related issues, audits, and penalties.

5. Real-Time Reporting and Analytics:

Automated RCM systems generate real-time reports and analytics, providing insights into key performance indicators, financial metrics, and revenue cycle trends. This enables data-driven decision-making, performance monitoring, and proactive interventions to improve revenue cycle outcomes.

6. Improved Patient Satisfaction:

Automation streamlines patient registration, billing, and payment processes, enhancing the overall patient experience. It reduces paperwork, speeds up eligibility verification, and provides transparent billing information, leading to improved patient satisfaction.

7. Cost Reduction and Revenue Optimization:

RCM automation eliminates redundant processes, reduces administrative costs, and minimizes inefficiencies. It improves revenue capture, reduces denials, and optimizes reimbursement, leading to increased revenue for healthcare organizations.

Challenges of RCM Automation:

1. Initial Investment and Implementation:

Implementing RCM automation requires upfront investment in software, hardware, infrastructure, and staff training. Organizations must carefully assess their needs, budget constraints, and scalability requirements to ensure a successful implementation.

2. Data Integration and System Compatibility:

Integrating multiple systems and ensuring compatibility between EHR, RCM software, and other related systems can be complex. Data migration, system interfaces, and interoperability issues need to be addressed to enable seamless data flow across systems.

3. Change Management and Staff Training:

Automation introduces changes in processes, roles, and responsibilities, requiring staff training and change management initiatives. Proper training is crucial to ensure staff members are proficient in using the automated systems and adapting to new workflows.

4. System Complexity and Customization:

RCM automation systems can be complex, requiring customization to align with specific organizational needs. Organizations should assess their requirements and select systems that offer the flexibility to accommodate customization while maintaining usability.

5. Data Security and Privacy Concerns:

Automation involves the storage and transfer of sensitive patient data, raising concerns about data security and privacy. Healthcare organizations must implement robust security measures, ensure compliance with regulations like HIPAA, and regularly assess system vulnerabilities.

6. System Downtime and Technical Issues:

Automated systems may experience downtime or technical issues, which can disrupt revenue cycle operations. Organizations must have contingency plans in place to minimize the impact of system downtime and ensure prompt resolution of technical issues.

7. Staff Adoption and Resistance:

Some staff members may resist the adoption of automated systems due to concerns about job security, fear of technology, or lack of confidence in using new tools. Clear communication, training, and involving staff in the implementation process can help mitigate resistance.

Addressing these challenges through proper planning, stakeholder engagement, ongoing support, and continuous improvement efforts can contribute to successful RCM automation implementation. It is crucial for healthcare organizations to assess their unique needs, evaluate available solutions, and carefully plan the implementation process to leverage the benefits of RCM automation effectively.

Exercise 14: Technology and Automation in RCM

1. RCM Software and Systems Overview

Question 1: What is the role of RCM software in revenue cycle management (RCM)?

Answer: RCM software plays a crucial role in revenue cycle management by automating and streamlining various processes involved in the financial lifecycle of healthcare services. It enables efficient management of patient registration, claims submission, payment processing, denial management, and reporting. RCM software centralizes data, improves accuracy, enhances workflow efficiency, and provides insights for decision-making. It helps healthcare organizations optimize revenue collection, reduce administrative costs, and improve overall financial performance.

Question 2: What are some key features and functionalities of RCM software systems?

Answer: Some key features and functionalities of RCM software systems include:

- Patient registration and demographic data management

- Insurance verification and eligibility checking

- Claims generation, submission, and tracking

- Denial management and appeals processing

- Payment processing, including invoicing and payment posting

- Revenue analysis and reporting

- Integration with electronic health records (EHR) and other healthcare systems

- Compliance monitoring and auditing capabilities

- Financial performance analytics and KPI tracking

- Patient communication and engagement tools

- Scalability and adaptability to changing regulatory and industry requirements

2. Electronic Health Records (EHR) and Integration

Question 1: What is the role of electronic health records (EHR) in revenue cycle management (RCM)?

Answer: Electronic health records (EHR) play a vital role in revenue cycle management by providing a comprehensive and centralized repository of patient health information. Integration between EHR and RCM systems enables seamless data exchange and supports efficient revenue cycle processes. EHR integration facilitates accurate patient registration, documentation, coding, and billing. It enhances the accuracy of claims submission, reduces duplicate data entry, and improves overall operational efficiency in revenue cycle management.

Question 2: What are some benefits of integrating EHR with RCM systems?

Answer: Some benefits of integrating EHR with RCM systems include:

- Improved accuracy and efficiency in patient registration and demographic data management.

- Seamless transfer of coded data from EHR to RCM systems, reducing manual errors and improving claim accuracy.

- Real-time access to patient health information for eligibility verification and claim submission.

- Enhanced documentation and coding processes, ensuring proper reimbursement and reducing claim denials.

- Streamlined workflow and reduced administrative burden by eliminating duplicate data entry.

- Comprehensive view of patient information for informed decision-making and financial analysis.

- Simplified reporting and compliance with regulatory requirements.

- Improved patient satisfaction through streamlined processes and accurate billing.

3. Benefits and Challenges of RCM Automation

Question 1: What are some benefits of RCM automation in healthcare organizations?

Answer: Some benefits of RCM automation in healthcare organizations include:

- Increased operational efficiency and productivity through streamlined processes and reduced manual tasks.

- Improved accuracy in data entry, coding, and claims submission, leading to fewer errors and claim denials.

- Faster reimbursement cycles and reduced days in accounts receivable (DAR), enhancing cash flow.

- Enhanced financial performance and revenue optimization through better tracking, analysis, and reporting.

- Improved compliance with regulatory requirements and reduced risk of non-compliance.

- Better visibility into revenue cycle metrics, allowing for proactive decision-making and process improvements.

- Enhanced patient satisfaction through improved billing accuracy, clear communication, and efficient payment processing.

Question 2: What are some challenges organizations may face when implementing RCM automation?

Answer: Some challenges organizations may face when implementing RCM automation include:

- Initial financial investment in software implementation and infrastructure upgrades.

- Resistance to change from staff members accustomed to manual processes.

- Data integration challenges when integrating different systems or EHR platforms.

- Training and education of staff members on the new software and workflows.

- Ensuring data security and compliance with privacy regulations.

- Adapting to evolving technology and staying updated with industry changes.

- Potential disruption to workflow during the transition phase.

- Technical issues or software glitches that may impact productivity.

These exercises provide an opportunity to reinforce the knowledge gained from the chapter on Technology and Automation in RCM. The questions assess understanding and reinforce key concepts related to RCM software and systems, electronic health records (EHR) integration, and the benefits and challenges of RCM automation in revenue cycle management.

15. RCM Performance Measurement and Analysis

15.1 Key Performance Indicators (KPIs) for RCM:

Measuring and analyzing key performance indicators (KPIs) is essential for monitoring the effectiveness of revenue cycle management (RCM) processes and identifying areas for improvement. Here are some important KPIs that healthcare organizations can use to evaluate RCM performance:

1. Clean Claim Rate:

The clean claim rate measures the percentage of claims that are submitted to payers without errors or deficiencies. A higher clean claim rate indicates efficient billing and coding processes, leading to faster claim processing and reimbursement.

2. Days in Accounts Receivable (DAR):

DAR measures the average number of days it takes for a healthcare organization to collect payments after providing services. A lower DAR indicates improved cash flow and efficient accounts receivable management.

3. Denial Rate:

The denial rate calculates the percentage of claims that are denied by payers. A lower denial rate indicates effective claims management processes, accurate coding, and proper documentation, leading to higher reimbursement rates.

4. Collection Rate:

The collection rate measures the percentage of patient balances that are successfully collected. It reflects the effectiveness of patient billing and collections processes, as well as the organization's ability to collect patient payments.

5. First-Pass Payment Rate:

The first-pass payment rate measures the percentage of claims that are paid by payers on the first submission without requiring additional follow-up or appeals. A higher first-pass payment rate indicates efficient claims submission and reduces the need for rework or resubmission.

6. Accounts Receivable (AR) Aging:

AR aging categorizes outstanding balances by the length of time they have been unpaid. It helps assess the timeliness of payment collection and identifies areas of concern, such as a high proportion of overdue or unpaid balances.

7. Net Collection Rate:

The net collection rate measures the percentage of revenue collected after accounting for contractual adjustments, discounts, and write-offs. It provides insights into the organization's ability to maximize revenue capture and manage financial performance.

8. Cost to Collect:

Cost to collect measures the expenses incurred in the revenue cycle management process, including staff salaries, technology costs, and other related expenses. It helps assess the efficiency and cost-effectiveness of RCM operations.

9. Percentage of Payments by Payer Type:

This KPI breaks down payments received by payer type, such as Medicare, Medicaid, commercial insurance, and self-pay. It helps identify the organization's reliance on specific payers and the impact of payer mix on revenue.

10. Compliance Metrics:

Compliance metrics evaluate the organization's adherence to regulatory requirements and internal policies. These metrics may include the number of coding errors, audit findings, and compliance-related issues, helping identify areas for improvement in coding accuracy and documentation.

It's important to note that the selection of KPIs may vary based on the specific needs and goals of the healthcare organization. Regular tracking and analysis of these KPIs allow organizations to identify trends, set benchmarks, and implement targeted improvement strategies to optimize revenue cycle performance. Additionally, benchmarking against industry standards and peers can provide valuable insights into RCM effectiveness.

15.2 Reporting and Analytics for RCM:

Reporting and analytics are crucial components of revenue cycle management (RCM) as they provide valuable insights into the financial performance, operational efficiency, and key metrics of an organization's revenue cycle. Here are some important aspects of reporting and analytics for RCM:

1. Customized RCM Dashboards:

RCM dashboards consolidate key performance indicators (KPIs) and metrics into visual representations, providing a snapshot of the organization's revenue cycle health. Dashboards can be customized to display relevant metrics, trends, and benchmarks, allowing stakeholders to monitor performance at a glance.

2. Financial Performance Reports:

Financial performance reports provide a comprehensive overview of revenue cycle outcomes. These reports include metrics such as net revenue, gross charges, collections, bad debt, and contractual adjustments. They help analyze revenue trends, identify opportunities for improvement, and support financial decision-making.

3. Claim Performance Analysis:

Claim performance analysis focuses on the efficiency and accuracy of claims management processes. It examines metrics such as clean claim rate, first-pass payment rate, denial rate, and average reimbursement time. This analysis helps identify bottlenecks, areas for improvement, and strategies for reducing denials and improving reimbursement rates.

4. Accounts Receivable (AR) Aging Analysis:

AR aging analysis categorizes outstanding balances by the length of time they have been unpaid. This analysis enables organizations to monitor and address issues related to slow payment, identify trends in collection delays, and optimize accounts receivable management.

5. Denial Management Reports:

Denial management reports provide insights into the types, reasons, and patterns of claim denials. These reports help organizations understand the root causes of denials, track denial resolution efforts, and implement strategies to reduce denials and improve revenue recovery.

6. Coding Accuracy and Compliance Reports:

Coding accuracy and compliance reports assess the quality and compliance of coding practices. These reports identify coding errors, documentation gaps, and compliance-related issues, helping organizations improve coding accuracy, ensure compliance with regulations, and mitigate audit risks.

7. Patient Financial Performance Reports:

Patient financial performance reports analyze patient payment trends, collection rates, and outstanding balances. These reports help identify opportunities to optimize patient collections, enhance patient payment processes, and improve overall patient financial satisfaction.

8. Productivity and Efficiency Metrics:

Productivity and efficiency metrics focus on operational aspects of the revenue cycle, such as staff productivity, claim cycle time, and resource utilization. These metrics provide insights into operational bottlenecks, identify opportunities for workflow optimization, and support resource allocation decisions.

9. Revenue Cycle Forecasting:

Revenue cycle forecasting utilizes historical data, trend analysis, and predictive modeling techniques to project future revenue performance. It helps organizations anticipate revenue fluctuations, plan resource allocation, and identify potential revenue growth opportunities.

10. Ad Hoc Analysis and Drill-Down Capabilities:

Reporting and analytics tools should provide ad hoc analysis capabilities, allowing users to explore data, generate custom reports, and perform detailed drill-downs into specific metrics or segments. This flexibility enables in-depth analysis, anomaly detection, and identification of root causes.

Timely and accurate reporting, along with advanced analytics, enable healthcare organizations to monitor performance, identify trends, and take proactive measures to optimize their revenue cycle. Regular analysis and reporting provide the necessary insights to make informed decisions, implement targeted improvement strategies, and enhance financial outcomes.

15.3 Benchmarking and Continuous Improvement:

Benchmarking and continuous improvement are critical components of revenue cycle management (RCM) that enable healthcare organizations to assess their performance, identify areas for improvement, and implement strategies to optimize their revenue cycle processes. Here's an overview of benchmarking and continuous improvement in RCM:

1. Benchmarking:

Benchmarking involves comparing an organization's performance against industry standards, best practices, or peers. It provides a reference point for evaluating the effectiveness and efficiency of RCM processes. Key steps in benchmarking include:

a. Identify Metrics: Determine the key performance indicators (KPIs) relevant to RCM and select metrics for benchmarking, such as clean claim rate, denial rate, days in accounts receivable, or collection rate.

b. Data Collection: Collect relevant data from internal sources, industry databases, or benchmarking surveys. Ensure data accuracy and consistency across the benchmarked organizations.

c. Perform Analysis: Compare the organization's performance against benchmarks, identify performance gaps, and analyze the root causes of variations. This analysis helps pinpoint areas for improvement.

d. Set Targets: Establish realistic improvement targets based on benchmark data and organizational goals. These targets provide a reference point for measuring progress and driving continuous improvement efforts.

2. Continuous Improvement Process:

Continuous improvement is an ongoing effort to enhance RCM processes, optimize performance, and achieve better financial outcomes. It involves a systematic approach to identifying areas for improvement, implementing changes, and monitoring the results. Key steps in the continuous improvement process include:

a. Identify Improvement Opportunities: Analyze performance metrics, review benchmarking results, solicit feedback from stakeholders, and identify areas where RCM processes can be optimized or streamlined.

b. Establish Improvement Goals: Set specific, measurable, achievable, relevant, and time-bound (SMART) goals for each improvement opportunity. Align goals with organizational priorities and RCM objectives.

c. Implement Process Changes: Develop action plans to address improvement goals and implement process changes. This may involve modifying workflows, updating policies and procedures, providing additional training, or leveraging technology solutions.

d. Monitor and Measure: Continuously monitor the impact of process changes and measure the results against established goals and performance metrics. Collect feedback from staff members, patients, and other stakeholders to assess the effectiveness of the implemented changes.

e. Review and Adjust: Regularly review performance data, assess the outcomes of implemented changes, and identify further areas for refinement. Make adjustments to the improvement strategies as needed to maximize results.

f. Foster a Culture of Continuous Improvement: Encourage staff engagement and participation in the continuous improvement process. Foster a culture that values innovation, teamwork, and ongoing learning. Recognize and celebrate successes to sustain motivation and engagement.

3. Collaboration and Knowledge Sharing:

Engage key stakeholders, including RCM staff, clinical teams, and leadership, in the continuous improvement process. Encourage collaboration, share best practices, and learn from the experiences of others. Participate in industry forums, conferences, and networks to gain insights and stay updated on the latest trends and innovations in RCM.

4. Technology Enablement:

Leverage technology solutions, such as analytics tools, automation systems, and electronic health record (EHR) integration, to support benchmarking and continuous improvement efforts. These tools provide data visibility, automate processes, and enable data-driven decision-making to drive improvement initiatives.

5. Performance Monitoring and Reporting:

Regularly monitor performance metrics, track progress against benchmarks and improvement goals, and generate reports to communicate outcomes and share insights with key stakeholders. Use performance dashboards and analytics tools to provide real-time visibility into RCM performance.

By adopting a proactive approach to benchmarking and continuous improvement, healthcare organizations can enhance their revenue cycle performance, optimize financial outcomes, and adapt to evolving industry trends and challenges. The process should be iterative, with a focus on data-driven decision-making and a commitment to ongoing learning and innovation.

Exercise 15: RCM Performance Measurement and Analysis

1. Key Performance Indicators (KPIs) for RCM

Question 1: What are Key Performance Indicators (KPIs) in revenue cycle management (RCM), and why are they important?

Answer: Key Performance Indicators (KPIs) in RCM are measurable metrics used to evaluate the performance and effectiveness of revenue cycle processes. They provide insights into the financial health of an organization and help identify areas for improvement. KPIs are important because they enable organizations to monitor revenue cycle performance, set goals, track progress, and make data-driven decisions. They allow for comparisons over time, benchmarking against industry standards, and identifying opportunities for optimization and revenue enhancement.

Question 2: What are some examples of KPIs used in RCM?

Answer: Some examples of KPIs used in RCM include:

- Days in Accounts Receivable (DAR): Measures the average number of days it takes to collect payment after services are rendered.

- Clean Claims Rate: Calculates the percentage of claims submitted without errors or omissions that are accepted by payers on the first submission.

- Denial Rate: Measures the percentage of claims that are denied by payers.

- Net Collection Rate: Calculates the percentage of total billed charges that are collected after accounting for contractual adjustments, denials, and write-offs.

- First-Pass Payment Rate: Measures the percentage of claims that are paid by payers on the first submission.

- Cash Flow Cycle Time: Measures the time it takes from the date of service to the date of payment.

- Accounts Receivable (AR) Aging: Analyzes the distribution and aging of outstanding accounts receivable balances.

2. Reporting and Analytics for RCM

Question 1: What is the role of reporting and analytics in revenue cycle management (RCM)?

Answer: Reporting and analytics play a crucial role in RCM by providing meaningful insights and actionable information. They help organizations assess financial performance, identify trends, and make informed decisions. Reporting and analytics enable the monitoring of key metrics, identification of areas of improvement, and detection of potential issues or bottlenecks in revenue cycle processes. They support strategic planning, performance management, and data-driven decision-making to optimize revenue collection and enhance financial outcomes.

Question 2: What are some common types of reports and analytics used in RCM?

Answer: Some common types of reports and analytics used in RCM include:

- Financial Reports: Summarize revenue, collections, accounts receivable balances, and other financial metrics.

- Denial Analysis Reports: Identify patterns, reasons, and trends related to claim denials, helping organizations implement targeted denial management strategies.

- Aging Reports: Analyze outstanding accounts receivable balances by aging categories, helping organizations prioritize follow-up and collections efforts.

- Productivity Reports: Assess the efficiency and productivity of revenue cycle staff members and departments.

- Compliance Reports: Monitor adherence to regulatory requirements and compliance with internal policies and guidelines.

- Revenue Analysis and Forecasting: Project future revenue based on historical data and market trends.

- Benchmarking Reports: Compare key metrics against industry standards or peer organizations, identifying areas for improvement.

3. Benchmarking and Continuous Improvement

Question 1: What is benchmarking in revenue cycle management (RCM), and why is it important?

Answer: Benchmarking in RCM involves comparing an organization's performance against industry standards or best practices. It helps organizations assess their relative performance, identify gaps, and set targets for improvement. Benchmarking allows organizations to understand how they measure up against others, learn from successful practices, and identify areas for improvement. It fosters a culture of continuous improvement, encourages innovation, and helps organizations achieve optimal financial performance.

Question 2: How can organizations foster continuous improvement in revenue cycle management?

Answer: Organizations can foster continuous improvement in revenue cycle management by:

- Establishing a culture of performance improvement and embracing a mindset of continuous learning and growth.

- Conducting regular performance reviews and assessments to identify areas for improvement.

- Setting realistic goals and targets based on benchmarking and industry standards.

- Implementing process improvement initiatives, such as Lean or Six Sigma methodologies, to streamline workflows and eliminate waste.

- Encouraging staff engagement and involvement in identifying improvement opportunities and implementing changes.

- Utilizing data analytics and reporting to monitor performance, track progress, and identify opportunities for optimization.

- Implementing feedback loops and soliciting input from stakeholders to gather insights and suggestions for improvement.

- Investing in staff training and professional development to enhance skills and knowledge in revenue cycle management.

These exercises provide an opportunity to reinforce the knowledge gained from the chapter on RCM Performance Measurement and Analysis. The questions assess understanding and reinforce key concepts related to key performance indicators (KPIs) for RCM, reporting and analytics for RCM, and the importance of benchmarking and continuous improvement in revenue cycle management.

CASE STUDIES

1. Case Study: Streamlining Claims Submission Process

Description:

In this case study, we examine the journey of a healthcare organization that successfully implemented process improvements to streamline their claims submission process. The organization faced challenges with high claim denials, lengthy reimbursement cycles, and delayed cash flow. They recognized the need for efficiency and accuracy in claims submission to optimize revenue cycle management.

Challenges:

- High rate of claim denials leading to increased administrative burden and financial losses.

- Lengthy reimbursement cycles resulting in delayed cash flow and strained financial operations.

Strategies Implemented:

- Conducted a comprehensive analysis of claim denial reasons to identify common patterns and root causes.

- Developed standardized coding and documentation guidelines to ensure accurate and complete claim submission.

- Implemented training programs for physicians and coding staff to enhance coding proficiency and documentation accuracy.

- Introduced automated claim scrubbing tools to identify and rectify errors prior to submission.

- Enhanced communication and collaboration between clinical and administrative staff to address documentation gaps and ensure timely claim submission.

Measurable Outcomes:

- Significant reduction in claim denials by 30% within six months of implementing process improvements.

- Improved cash flow due to faster reimbursement cycles and timely payment posting.

- Increased revenue capture by minimizing coding and billing errors.

- Enhanced staff productivity and morale through streamlined processes and reduced rework.

2. Case Study: Implementing RCM Automation in a Hospital Setting

Description:

This case study explores the journey of a hospital that implemented revenue cycle management automation to improve operational efficiency and financial performance. The organization recognized the need for streamlined processes, reduced manual tasks, and increased accuracy in revenue-related workflows.

Challenges:

- Manual and paper-based processes leading to inefficiencies, errors, and delays in revenue cycle operations.

- Lack of visibility into key revenue cycle metrics and performance indicators.

- Inconsistent workflows and disjointed communication between departments.

Strategies Implemented:

- Conducted a thorough assessment of existing processes to identify areas for automation.

- Selected a comprehensive RCM software system that integrated with existing EHR and billing systems.

- Customized the software to align with organizational workflows and requirements.

- Trained staff members on using the new system and provided ongoing support and education.

- Implemented automated workflows for patient registration, claims submission, denial management, and reporting.

Measurable Outcomes:

- Streamlined processes, reduced manual tasks, and eliminated paper-based workflows.

- Increased accuracy in coding, documentation, and claims submission.

- Improved cash flow and reduced days in accounts receivable (DAR) by 20%.

- Enhanced reporting and analytics capabilities, enabling data-driven decision-making.

- Higher staff productivity, improved collaboration, and reduced administrative burden.

3. Case Study: Improving Denial Management and Appeals Process

Description:

This case study focuses on a healthcare organization that revamped their denial management and appeals process to optimize revenue cycle management. The organization faced challenges with high denial rates, delayed reimbursements, and revenue leakage due to ineffective denial management practices.

Challenges:

- High rate of claim denials resulting in revenue loss and increased administrative costs.

- Inefficient denial management and appeals process leading to delayed reimbursement and revenue leakage.

- Lack of standardized workflows and communication protocols for denial resolution.

Strategies Implemented:

- Conducted a comprehensive analysis of denial reasons and patterns to identify common issues.

- Developed a centralized denial management and appeals team to ensure timely resolution.

- Implemented technology solutions for denial tracking, workflow management, and reporting.

- Established clear communication channels between clinical and administrative staff for denial resolution.

- Conducted training programs for staff members on denial prevention, effective appeals, and regulatory compliance.

Measurable Outcomes:

- Significant reduction in claim denial rates by 40% within one year of implementing the new process.

- Improved denial resolution time, leading to faster reimbursement cycles.

- Increased revenue capture by successfully appealing denied claims.

- Enhanced collaboration and communication between departments, resulting in streamlined workflows.

- Improved financial performance and reduced revenue leakage.

4. Case Study: Enhancing Patient Collections and Financial Assistance Programs

Description:

This case study showcases a healthcare organization's efforts to improve patient collections and enhance their financial assistance programs. The organization recognized the importance of clear and transparent billing practices, flexible payment options, and effective communication to enhance patient satisfaction and maximize revenue collection.

Challenges:

- High rate of patient bad debt and uncollected balances.

- Inadequate patient education and communication regarding financial responsibilities.

- Limited flexibility in payment options and financial assistance programs.

Strategies Implemented:

- Implemented patient-centric billing practices, such as clear and transparent statements with itemized charges.

- Enhanced patient communication regarding financial responsibilities, payment options, and available financial assistance programs.

- Provided financial counseling and support to help patients understand their obligations and explore available resources.

- Developed flexible payment plans tailored to patients' financial capabilities.

- Strengthened collaboration with payers and government programs to maximize financial assistance eligibility and reimbursement.

Measurable Outcomes:

- Improved patient satisfaction scores related to billing and financial interactions.

- Reduced patient bad debt and uncollected balances by implementing proactive collection strategies.

- Increased patient payment compliance through flexible payment options and financial counseling.

- Enhanced utilization of financial assistance programs, leading to increased reimbursement.

- Improved financial performance through higher collection rates and reduced write-offs.

These elaborated case studies provide practical examples, facts, and samples to demonstrate the challenges faced by healthcare organizations and the strategies implemented to achieve positive outcomes in revenue cycle management. Including these detailed case studies in the comprehensive guide will provide students with valuable insights into real-world scenarios and help them understand the practical application of revenue cycle management concepts.

FINAL TEST

Section 1: Revenue Cycle Fundamentals

1. What is the primary objective of revenue cycle management (RCM)?

2. List and briefly explain the key components of the revenue cycle.

3. Define the following terms:
   a) Accounts Receivable (AR)
   b) Explanation of Benefits (EOB)
   c) Remittance Advice (RA)
   d) Clean Claim

4. Differentiate between fee-for-service and value-based reimbursement models.

5. Explain the significance of revenue cycle management in healthcare organizations.

Section 2: Revenue Cycle Planning and Implementation

6. Discuss the importance of setting goals and objectives in revenue cycle management planning.

7. Outline the steps involved in assessing organizational readiness for implementing RCM.

8. Explain the key considerations when developing an RCM implementation strategy.

9. Define change management and discuss its role in successful RCM implementation.

Section 3: Patient Registration and Pre-Service Revenue Cycle

10. Describe the importance of accurate patient pre-registration and demographic data collection.

11. Discuss the process of insurance verification and eligibility checking.

12. Explain the concept of patient financial responsibility and the importance of estimation.

Section 4: Scheduling and Patient Access Management

13. Discuss efficient appointment scheduling strategies in healthcare organizations.

14. Outline the best practices for patient access management to improve operational efficiency.

15. Explain strategies for reducing no-shows and cancellations in healthcare settings.

Section 5: Medical Coding and Documentation

16. Define the medical coding systems CPT, ICD, and HCPCS, and explain their significance in RCM.

17. Describe accurate documentation and coding guidelines in healthcare.

18. Discuss the role of risk adjustment coding in revenue cycle management.

Section 6: Charge Capture and Reimbursement

19. Explain the importance of charge capture in revenue cycle management.

20. Outline the documentation and coding requirements for proper charge capture.

21. Discuss different reimbursement methodologies and rates in healthcare.

Section 7: Claims Submission and Adjudication

22. Describe the claims submission process and the key requirements for successful claim submission.

23. Explain the principles and best practices for clean claims submission.

24. Discuss the process of payer adjudication and the analysis of claim rejections.

Section 8: Denial Management and Appeals

25. Identify common causes of claim denials and explain their impact on revenue cycle management.

26. Discuss denial prevention and resolution strategies to minimize claim denials.

27. Explain the steps involved in an effective appeal process to maximize reimbursement.

Section 9: Insurance Follow-Up and Accounts Receivable Management

28. Describe the process of monitoring unpaid claims and utilizing aging reports.

29. Discuss timely and effective follow-up strategies for insurance claims.

30. Explain methods for reducing Days in Accounts Receivable (DAR) in healthcare organizations.

Section 10: Patient Billing and Collections

31. Provide an overview of the patient billing cycle in revenue cycle management.

32. Discuss the importance of clear and transparent patient statements.

33. Outline patient collections strategies and the role of financial assistance programs.

Section 11: Financial Assistance and Charity Care

34. Describe the overview of financial assistance programs in healthcare organizations.

35. Explain the eligibility criteria and the application process for financial assistance programs.

36. Discuss the compliance requirements associated with financial assistance programs.

Section 12: Healthcare Compliance and Regulatory Considerations

37. Discuss the importance of HIPAA in healthcare compliance and patient data privacy.

38. Explain the implications of anti-fraud and abuse regulations, such as the Stark Law and False Claims Act, on revenue cycle management.

39. Describe the process of RCM compliance audits and monitoring.

Section 13: Technology and Automation in RCM

40. Discuss the overview of RCM software and systems in revenue cycle management.

41. Explain the role of electronic health records (EHR) and their integration in RCM.

42. Outline the benefits and challenges of RCM automation in healthcare organizations.

Section 14: RCM Performance Measurement and Analysis

43. Identify key performance indicators (KPIs) for revenue cycle management and explain their significance.

44. Discuss the importance of reporting and analytics in revenue cycle management.

45. Explain the concept of benchmarking and its role in continuous improvement.

Answer Key:

1. The primary objective of revenue cycle management is to optimize the financial performance of healthcare organizations by effectively managing the financial lifecycle of patient care.

2. Key components of the revenue cycle include patient registration, scheduling, coding, charge capture, claims submission, payment processing, denial management, and accounts receivable management.

3.

a) Accounts Receivable (AR): The outstanding balances owed to a healthcare organization for services rendered.

b) Explanation of Benefits (EOB): A document provided by the insurance company detailing the coverage and payment information for a specific claim.

c) Remittance Advice (RA): A document provided by the payer that explains the payment details for a claim.

d) Clean Claim: A claim that is complete, accurate, and meets all the requirements for timely processing and reimbursement.

4. Fee-for-service reimbursement is based on the quantity of services provided, while value-based reimbursement focuses on the quality and outcomes of care provided.

5. Revenue cycle management is crucial in healthcare organizations as it ensures timely and accurate reimbursement, improves cash flow, reduces claim denials, enhances operational efficiency, and supports financial sustainability.

6. Setting goals and objectives in revenue cycle management planning helps organizations align their efforts, establish benchmarks for success, and track progress towards achieving desired outcomes.

7. Assessing organizational readiness involves evaluating the current state of revenue cycle processes, technology infrastructure, staff capabilities, and stakeholder buy-in to determine the organization's preparedness for RCM implementation.

8. Developing an RCM implementation strategy requires defining project goals, establishing timelines and milestones, allocating resources, selecting appropriate technology solutions, and designing workflows that align with organizational needs.

9. Change management involves managing the human side of RCM implementation, including addressing resistance to change, engaging stakeholders, providing training and support, and fostering a culture of adaptability and continuous improvement.

10. Accurate patient pre-registration and demographic data collection are essential to ensure correct patient identification, insurance verification, and efficient billing processes. It helps prevent claim denials and reduces administrative errors.

11. Insurance verification and eligibility checking involve verifying a patient's insurance coverage, confirming their eligibility for services, and understanding their benefits and coverage limitations. This process helps ensure accurate billing and prevents claim rejections or underpayment.

12. Patient financial responsibility refers to the portion of healthcare costs that patients are responsible for paying out-of-pocket. Estimation of patient financial responsibility helps patients understand their financial obligations and facilitates upfront payment or the establishment of payment plans.

13. Efficient appointment scheduling strategies aim to maximize provider utilization, minimize wait times, and improve patient satisfaction. These strategies may include optimizing appointment templates, streamlining referral processes, and using technology to facilitate scheduling.

14. Patient access management best practices focus on optimizing the patient intake process, including registration, insurance verification, and ensuring a smooth transition into care. This involves implementing standardized workflows, leveraging technology for data capture, and providing staff training on patient-centric interactions.

15. Strategies for reducing no-shows and cancellations include appointment reminders, patient education on the importance of keeping appointments, optimizing scheduling processes to reduce wait times, and implementing policies and incentives to encourage adherence to appointments.

16. CPT (Current Procedural Terminology), ICD (International Classification of Diseases), and HCPCS (Healthcare Common Procedure Coding System) are coding systems used in healthcare to classify and document medical procedures, diagnoses, and supplies. These coding systems are essential for accurate billing, reimbursement, and data analysis.

17. Accurate documentation and coding guidelines ensure that medical services and procedures are properly documented, coded, and billed. This includes capturing all relevant information, using appropriate codes, and complying with coding guidelines to support accurate and appropriate reimbursement.

18. Risk adjustment coding involves capturing additional diagnostic codes to reflect the complexity and severity of a patient's condition. It helps ensure appropriate reimbursement for patients with more complex medical needs and supports accurate risk assessment and prediction.

19. Charge capture is the process of accurately capturing and recording the services and procedures provided to patients for billing purposes. It ensures that all services rendered are appropriately documented and billed to the payer.

20. Documentation and coding requirements for proper charge capture include capturing all billable services, accurately documenting diagnoses and procedures, following coding guidelines and conventions, and ensuring documentation supports the level of service provided.

21. Reimbursement methodologies and rates vary based on payer type and contracts. Common reimbursement methods include fee-for-service, bundled payments, capitation, and value-based arrangements. Rates may be negotiated with payers or set by regulatory bodies.

22. The claims submission process involves preparing and submitting claims to payers for reimbursement. Key requirements include accurate patient and provider information, coding compliance, proper claim form completion, and timely submission.

23. Clean claim principles include submitting accurate and complete claims on the first submission, ensuring all required information is included, adhering to payer-specific guidelines, and following coding and billing rules.

24. Payer adjudication involves the evaluation and processing of claims by payers to determine reimbursement. Analysis of claim rejections involves identifying the reasons for claim denials, analyzing trends, and implementing corrective actions to prevent future denials.

25. Common causes of claim denials include coding errors, lack of medical necessity, incomplete documentation, eligibility issues, and billing errors. Claim denials impact revenue cycle management by delaying reimbursement and increasing administrative costs.

26. Denial prevention and resolution strategies involve proactive measures such as accurate documentation, staff education, claims scrubbing, and implementing effective denial management processes. Resolving denials requires timely investigation, clear communication, and filing appeals when necessary.

27. An effective appeal process involves understanding denial reasons, gathering supporting documentation, preparing a strong appeal letter, and following the payer's appeals process. Maximizing reimbursement involves identifying opportunities for overturning denials and recovering rightful reimbursement.

28. Monitoring unpaid claims and utilizing aging reports involves regularly reviewing outstanding claims, identifying overdue payments, and prioritizing follow-up activities. This helps to ensure timely reimbursement and reduces the risk of accounts becoming uncollectible.

29. Timely and effective follow-up strategies for insurance claims include establishing follow-up timelines, leveraging technology for claim tracking, utilizing denial management workflows, and maintaining open communication with payers to resolve outstanding issues.

30. Reducing Days in Accounts Receivable (DAR) involves implementing strategies to accelerate cash flow and minimize the time it takes to convert billed services into collected payments. This may include streamlining billing processes, optimizing claims submission, and implementing effective accounts receivable management practices.

31. The patient billing cycle encompasses the entire process of generating and delivering patient bills, including statement generation, payment posting, and patient communication. It involves ensuring accurate billing, providing clear and concise statements, and facilitating timely payment collection.

32. Clear and transparent patient statements are essential for effective communication of financial obligations. They should provide detailed information about services rendered, charges, insurance coverage, patient responsibility, payment options, and contact details for billing inquiries.

33. Patient collections strategies involve implementing various methods to collect patient balances, such as setting up payment plans, offering online payment options, providing financial counseling, and employing collection agencies when necessary. Financial assistance programs can also help patients who are unable to afford their medical expenses.

34. Financial assistance programs aim to provide support to patients who are unable to pay for their medical expenses. These programs may include charity care, sliding fee scales, Medicaid, and other forms of financial assistance based on income eligibility.

35. Eligibility criteria for financial assistance programs typically depend on income levels, household size, and other factors. The application process may involve completing an application form, providing supporting documents, and undergoing a financial assessment.

36. Compliance with regulatory requirements for financial assistance programs involves ensuring adherence to applicable laws and regulations, such as the Affordable Care Act (ACA) and state-specific guidelines. This includes maintaining accurate records, providing appropriate disclosures, and following non-discrimination policies.

37. HIPAA (Health Insurance Portability and Accountability Act) is a federal law that protects the privacy and security of patient health information. It sets standards for the use, disclosure, and safeguarding of protected health information (PHI) in healthcare organizations.

38. Anti-fraud and abuse regulations, such as the Stark Law and False Claims Act, are designed to prevent fraudulent billing practices and improper financial relationships in healthcare. These regulations impose restrictions on referrals, prohibit certain billing practices, and impose penalties for violations.

39. RCM compliance audits and monitoring involve conducting regular assessments of revenue cycle processes, documentation, coding practices, and adherence to regulatory guidelines. This helps identify areas of non-compliance and implement corrective actions to mitigate risks.

40. RCM software and systems overview provides an understanding of the different types of software solutions available for revenue cycle management. This includes practice management systems, electronic health records (EHR), billing and coding software, and revenue cycle management platforms.

41. Electronic Health Records (EHR) integration in revenue cycle management involves the seamless exchange of patient information between clinical and financial systems. This integration improves data accuracy, reduces manual entry errors, and enhances billing efficiency.

42. The benefits of RCM automation include increased accuracy in billing and coding, streamlined workflows, reduced administrative burden, improved claim submission and processing, enhanced revenue capture, and improved data analytics capabilities. Challenges may include initial implementation costs and the need for staff training and system integration.

43. Key Performance Indicators (KPIs) for revenue cycle management are metrics used to measure the performance and efficiency of revenue cycle operations. Examples include days in accounts receivable (DAR), clean claim rate, denial rate, and collection rate.

44. Reporting and analytics play a crucial role in revenue cycle management by providing insights into key performance indicators, claim metrics, denial trends, and financial performance. This data helps organizations identify areas for improvement, make informed decisions, and track progress towards goals.

45. Benchmarking involves comparing an organization's revenue cycle performance against industry standards or best practices. It helps identify areas of strength and areas that require improvement, enabling organizations to set performance targets and continuously improve their revenue cycle operations.

APPENDIX

1. Glossary of RCM Terminologies: A comprehensive list of commonly used terms and acronyms in revenue cycle management.

Below is a sample glossary of commonly used terms and acronyms in revenue cycle management (RCM):

1. Accounts Receivable (AR): The amount of money owed to a healthcare organization for services rendered but not yet collected.

2. Clean Claim: A claim that is complete, accurate, and free of errors or deficiencies, allowing for smooth processing and timely reimbursement.

3. Claim Denial: The rejection of a submitted claim by a payer due to various reasons, such as coding errors, missing information, or lack of medical necessity.

4. CPT (Current Procedural Terminology): A coding system developed by the American Medical Association (AMA) used to describe medical procedures and services performed by healthcare providers.

5. Days in Accounts Receivable (DAR): The average number of days it takes for a healthcare organization to collect payments after providing services.

6. EHR (Electronic Health Record): A digital record that contains patient health information, including medical history, diagnoses, treatments, and test results.

7. ICD (International Classification of Diseases): A coding system used to classify and code diagnoses, symptoms, and procedures for medical billing and reporting purposes.

8. Payer: An entity, such as an insurance company or government program, that provides payment for healthcare services.

9. Pre-authorization: The process of obtaining approval from a payer before providing certain medical services or procedures to ensure coverage and reimbursement.

10. Revenue Cycle: The entire process of capturing, managing, and collecting revenue for healthcare services, starting from patient registration to final payment.

11. RCM (Revenue Cycle Management): The strategic management of all administrative and clinical functions related to the capture, management, and collection of revenue for healthcare services.

12. Remittance Advice: A document provided by a payer that explains the payment made for a claim, including details of any adjustments, denials, or additional information.

13. Self-Pay: Refers to patients who do not have insurance coverage and are responsible for paying for their healthcare services out of pocket.

14. UB-04: The standard claim form used for submitting institutional healthcare claims, including those from hospitals, nursing homes, and other healthcare facilities.

15. Unbilled Services: Services provided by healthcare providers that have not yet been billed to the payer or patient.

Please note that this glossary is not exhaustive and can be expanded based on specific needs and industry variations.

Here are some recommended books on revenue cycle management (RCM) that provide in-depth knowledge and insights:

1. "The Healthcare Revenue Cycle: Financial Management Strategies" by Anne McLeod and James W. O'Connell

   This comprehensive book covers all aspects of the revenue cycle, including billing, coding, reimbursement, denials management, and financial reporting. It offers practical strategies for optimizing revenue cycle performance.

2. "Revenue Cycle Management Best Practices: Optimizing the Healthcare Revenue Cycle" by Duane C. Abbey

   Duane C. Abbey, a renowned expert in healthcare reimbursement, provides a comprehensive guide to optimizing revenue cycle management. The book covers topics such as charge capture, coding, claims processing, denials management, and compliance.

3. "Principles of Healthcare Revenue Cycle" by Elizabeth H. Woodcock

   This book offers a practical approach to revenue cycle management, covering topics such as registration, eligibility verification, coding, billing, denials management, and financial performance analysis. It includes case studies and real-world examples to illustrate key concepts.

4. "The Physician Billing Process: Avoiding Potholes in the Road to Getting Paid" by Marty Kotlar

   Written specifically for physicians and medical practices, this book focuses on the billing process, coding, and documentation requirements. It provides practical tips for improving billing efficiency, reducing denials, and maximizing revenue.

5. "Revenue Cycle Management Toolkit: A Comprehensive Guide for Healthcare Organizations" by Loretta L. Manning

   This toolkit-style book offers a step-by-step approach to revenue cycle management, covering topics such as front-end processes, coding, claims submission, denials management, payment posting, and collections. It includes practical tools, templates, and checklists.

6. "The Financially Intelligent Physician: What They Didn't Teach You in Medical School" by David K. Nartonis

   While not focused solely on RCM, this book provides valuable insights into financial management for physicians. It covers topics such as revenue generation, practice financial analysis, managing expenses, and improving profitability.

These books offer a wealth of knowledge and practical guidance for professionals involved in revenue cycle management in healthcare organizations. They can help deepen understanding, enhance performance, and provide strategies for overcoming challenges in the complex healthcare reimbursement landscape.

Here is a compilation of reputable online courses and training programs focused on revenue cycle management (RCM), available on platforms like Udemy, Coursera, and LinkedIn Learning:

1. Udemy:

  - "Revenue Cycle Management Fundamentals" by Lindsey Morse: This course provides a comprehensive overview of RCM, covering topics such as billing, coding, claims management, denials management, and financial reporting.

  - "Optimizing the Revenue Cycle" by Timothy Hoffmann: This course explores strategies for optimizing the revenue cycle, including topics like charge capture, coding accuracy, denials prevention, and improving financial performance.

2. Coursera:

  - "Healthcare Finance and Financial Management" by University of Pennsylvania: This course covers financial management principles in healthcare organizations, including revenue cycle management, reimbursement systems, and healthcare economics.

  - "Revenue Cycle Management in Healthcare" by University of Miami: This course focuses on the key components of revenue cycle management, including patient access, billing, coding, claims processing, denials management, and financial reporting.

3. LinkedIn Learning:

  - "Revenue Cycle Management: Patient Access" by Elizabeth Woods: This course provides insights into patient access processes in the revenue cycle, including topics like registration, insurance verification, eligibility, and upfront payment collections.

  - "Healthcare Billing and Revenue Cycle Management" by George Washington University: This course covers the fundamentals of healthcare billing and revenue cycle management, including coding, claims processing, denials management, and compliance.

These online courses offer flexibility in terms of self-paced learning and are designed to provide comprehensive knowledge and practical skills in revenue cycle management. It's recommended to review the course syllabus, duration, and user reviews before selecting a course that aligns with your specific learning goals and preferences.

4. Professional Associations and Organizations: A list of industry associations and organizations dedicated to revenue cycle management. Include links to their websites for further information and resources.

Here is a list of professional associations and organizations dedicated to revenue cycle management (RCM), along with links to their websites for further information and resources:

1. Healthcare Financial Management Association (HFMA):

  Website: https://www.hfma.org/

  HFMA is a leading professional association for healthcare finance and revenue cycle professionals. It offers educational resources, certification programs, networking opportunities, and industry insights.

2. American Association of Healthcare Administrative Management (AAHAM):

  Website: https://www.aaham.org/

  AAHAM is a national professional association focused on healthcare administrative management. It provides education, certification, advocacy, and networking opportunities for revenue cycle professionals.

3. Medical Group Management Association (MGMA):

  Website: https://www.mgma.com/

  MGMA is a professional association for medical practice management professionals. It offers resources, networking, and education on various topics, including revenue cycle management.

4. Healthcare Information and Management Systems Society (HIMSS):

  Website: https://www.himss.org/

  HIMSS is a global organization focused on healthcare information and technology. It provides resources, events, and networking opportunities related to revenue cycle management and health IT.

5. American Health Information Management Association (AHIMA):

  Website: https://www.ahima.org/

AHIMA is a professional association for health information management professionals. It offers resources, certifications, and educational programs related to coding, documentation, and revenue cycle management.

6. Healthcare Billing and Management Association (HBMA):

Website: https://www.hbma.org/

HBMA is an association for revenue cycle management professionals in the medical billing and coding industry. It provides educational resources, networking opportunities, and industry advocacy.

These professional associations and organizations offer valuable resources, educational programs, networking opportunities, and industry updates for revenue cycle management professionals. It is recommended to explore their websites and consider becoming a member to access their full range of benefits and resources.

5. Industry Publications and Journals: A selection of relevant publications and journals that cover topics related to revenue cycle management. Include both print and online publications.

Here is a selection of relevant publications and journals that cover topics related to revenue cycle management (RCM). Please note that availability may vary between print and online formats:

1. Journal of Healthcare Finance:

   Website: https://www.healthcarefinancials.com/

   This journal focuses on financial management and healthcare finance, covering topics related to RCM, reimbursement, financial analysis, and revenue optimization.

2. Healthcare Financial Management:

   Website: https://www.hfma.org/leadership/hfm/

   Published by the Healthcare Financial Management Association (HFMA), this publication provides in-depth coverage of healthcare finance and RCM topics, including best practices, industry trends, and case studies.

3. Medical Practice Management:

   Website: https://www.mgma.com/publications/medical-practice-management

   Published by the Medical Group Management Association (MGMA), this magazine covers various aspects of medical practice management, including RCM, billing, coding, compliance, and operational efficiency.

4. Journal of AHIMA (American Health Information Management Association):

   Website: https://www.ahima.org/publications/journal/

   This journal focuses on health information management, including coding, documentation, and RCM topics. It provides insights into regulatory updates, best practices, and emerging trends.

5. Revenue Cycle Strategist:

   Website: https://www.rcmstrategist.com/

This publication offers insights and best practices for revenue cycle professionals. It covers topics such as denials management, billing strategies, coding updates, compliance, and revenue cycle technology.

6. Becker's Hospital Review:

Website: https://www.beckershospitalreview.com/

Becker's Hospital Review provides industry news, insights, and analysis on various healthcare topics, including revenue cycle management, billing, and reimbursement.

7. Healthcare Business Monthly:

Website: https://www.aapc.com/medical-coding-books/healthcare-business-monthly.aspx

Published by the American Academy of Professional Coders (AAPC), this magazine covers topics related to coding, billing, and RCM, providing practical guidance and industry updates.

These publications and journals offer a wealth of information, best practices, case studies, and industry updates for revenue cycle management professionals. It is recommended to explore their websites for access to articles, subscription details, and additional resources.

6. Websites and Blogs: Links to websites and blogs that offer valuable resources, articles, and industry updates on revenue cycle management.

Here are some websites and blogs that offer valuable resources, articles, and industry updates on revenue cycle management (RCM):

1. RevCycleIntelligence:

   Website: https://revcycleintelligence.com/

   RevCycleIntelligence provides news, articles, and insights on various aspects of revenue cycle management, including billing, coding, reimbursement, technology, and regulatory updates.

2. Becker's Hospital Review:

   Website: https://www.beckershospitalreview.com/finance/revenue-cycle-management.html

   Becker's Hospital Review offers a dedicated section on revenue cycle management, featuring articles, interviews, and expert insights on RCM trends, strategies, and best practices.

3. Healthcare Financial Management Association (HFMA):

   Website: https://www.hfma.org/

   The HFMA website provides resources, articles, webinars, and industry updates on revenue cycle management, financial management, and healthcare finance.

4. Revenue Cycle Insights:

   Website: https://www.revenuecycleinsights.org/

   Revenue Cycle Insights offers articles, case studies, and resources on revenue cycle management, with a focus on healthcare finance, billing, coding, and reimbursement.

5. Change Healthcare Blog:

   Website: https://www.changehealthcare.com/blog

   The Change Healthcare blog covers various topics related to revenue cycle management, including payment innovation, technology solutions, regulatory updates, and industry trends.

6. MGMA Insights Blog:

  Website: https://www.mgma.com/data/data-stories/mgma-insights-blog

  The MGMA Insights Blog features articles, industry updates, and expert perspectives on revenue cycle management, medical practice management, and healthcare trends.

7. AAPC Blog:

  Website: https://www.aapc.com/blog/

  The AAPC blog covers topics related to coding, billing, compliance, and revenue cycle management, providing insights, tips, and news relevant to RCM professionals.

8. Healthcare Finance News:

  Website: https://www.healthcarefinancenews.com/

  Healthcare Finance News offers articles, industry updates, and thought leadership on healthcare finance, including revenue cycle management and financial performance.

These websites and blogs provide a wealth of resources, articles, and industry updates on revenue cycle management. They are great sources to stay informed, access expert insights, and keep up with the latest trends and best practices in RCM.

7. Software and Technology Solutions: An overview of popular revenue cycle management software and technology solutions. Include brief descriptions and links to their websites for further exploration.

Here is an overview of popular revenue cycle management (RCM) software and technology solutions that are widely used in the healthcare industry:

1. Epic Systems Corporation:

   Website: https://www.epic.com/

   Epic offers a comprehensive suite of RCM solutions, including billing, claims management, patient access, and revenue optimization. Their software integrates with electronic health records (EHR) systems and provides end-to-end revenue cycle management capabilities.

2. Cerner Corporation:

   Website: https://www.cerner.com/

   Cerner offers RCM solutions that encompass the entire revenue cycle, from patient registration to payment. Their software includes features such as coding, claims management, denials management, and financial reporting.

3. NextGen Healthcare:

   Website: https://www.nextgen.com/

   NextGen Healthcare offers a range of RCM solutions tailored for medical practices, including billing, coding, claims management, and patient collections. Their software focuses on streamlining workflows and improving revenue cycle efficiency.

4. Allscripts Healthcare Solutions:

   Website: https://www.allscripts.com/

   Allscripts provides RCM solutions that integrate with their EHR platforms, offering features such as billing, coding, claims management, and denials management. Their software aims to improve revenue capture and accelerate reimbursement.

5. eClinicalWorks:

Website: https://www.eclinicalworks.com/

eClinicalWorks offers RCM solutions that encompass the entire patient lifecycle, including appointment scheduling, registration, coding, claims management, and patient billing. Their software focuses on optimizing revenue and enhancing patient financial experience.

6. Meditech:

Website: https://ehr.meditech.com/

Meditech offers RCM solutions that integrate with their EHR platform, providing features such as billing, coding, claims management, and financial reporting. Their software aims to streamline revenue cycle processes and improve financial performance.

7. Athenahealth:

Website: https://www.athenahealth.com/

Athenahealth offers cloud-based RCM solutions that cover patient registration, claims management, billing, and financial reporting. Their software focuses on automation, revenue optimization, and improving the patient financial experience.

8. Greenway Health:

Website: https://www.greenwayhealth.com/

Greenway Health provides RCM solutions for ambulatory practices, offering features such as coding, claims management, denial management, and financial reporting. Their software aims to enhance revenue cycle efficiency and maximize collections.

Please note that the availability and suitability of software solutions may vary based on the specific needs and requirements of healthcare organizations. It is recommended to visit the respective websites for detailed information, demos, and to request pricing based on your organization's specific needs.

8. Compliance and Regulatory Resources: Links to regulatory websites, such as the Centers for Medicare and Medicaid Services (CMS) and the Office for Civil Rights (OCR), providing access to guidelines, regulations, and updates related to revenue cycle management compliance.

Here are links to regulatory websites and resources that provide access to guidelines, regulations, and updates related to revenue cycle management compliance:

1. Centers for Medicare and Medicaid Services (CMS):

  Website: https://www.cms.gov/

  CMS is a federal agency within the U.S. Department of Health and Human Services (HHS) that administers the Medicare and Medicaid programs. Their website offers a wealth of resources, guidelines, regulations, and updates related to reimbursement, coding, billing, and compliance.

2. Office of Inspector General (OIG):

  Website: https://oig.hhs.gov/

  The OIG is an independent agency within the HHS that promotes efficiency, effectiveness, and integrity in the administration of HHS programs. Their website provides access to various resources, including compliance guidance, advisory opinions, and fraud alerts.

3. Office for Civil Rights (OCR):

  Website: https://www.hhs.gov/hipaa/for-professionals/index.html

  The OCR is responsible for enforcing federal regulations related to the privacy and security of protected health information (PHI) under the Health Insurance Portability and Accountability Act (HIPAA). Their website offers guidance, regulations, and resources on HIPAA compliance.

4. American Medical Association (AMA):

  Website: https://www.ama-assn.org/

  The AMA is a professional association for physicians and offers resources related to coding, billing, reimbursement, and compliance. Their website provides access to coding guidelines, CPT updates, and other resources relevant to revenue cycle management.

5. American Health Information Management Association (AHIMA):

  Website: https://www.ahima.org/

  AHIMA is a professional association for health information management professionals. Their website offers resources, guidelines, and updates related to coding, documentation, privacy, and compliance.

6. National Correct Coding Initiative (NCCI):

  Website: https://www.cms.gov/Medicare/Coding/NationalCorrectCodInitEd

  NCCI is an initiative by CMS that promotes correct coding methodologies and edits to prevent improper coding and billing. The NCCI website provides access to coding policies, guidelines, and edits that impact the revenue cycle.

It's important to regularly visit these websites to stay updated on the latest regulations, guidelines, and compliance requirements related to revenue cycle management. Additionally, healthcare organizations should consult legal and compliance professionals to ensure adherence to all applicable regulations and requirements.

9. Professional Certification Programs: Information about recognized professional certifications in revenue cycle management, such as Certified Revenue Cycle Professional (CRCP) and Certified Professional Biller (CPB). Include details on eligibility criteria and certification bodies.

Here is information about recognized professional certifications in revenue cycle management (RCM):

1. Certified Revenue Cycle Professional (CRCP):

Certification Body: Healthcare Financial Management Association (HFMA)

Website: https://www.hfma.org/certification/

The CRCP certification is offered by HFMA and is designed for revenue cycle professionals who demonstrate expertise in various aspects of RCM. It covers topics such as revenue cycle fundamentals, patient access, billing, claims management, and financial reporting. Eligibility criteria, exam details, and study resources can be found on the HFMA website.

2. Certified Professional Biller (CPB):

Certification Body: American Academy of Professional Coders (AAPC)

Website: https://www.aapc.com/certification/cpb/

The CPB certification is offered by AAPC and focuses specifically on the billing aspect of the revenue cycle. It validates proficiency in medical billing processes, including coding, claims submission, payment posting, and compliance. The AAPC website provides information on eligibility requirements, exam details, and study resources for the CPB certification.

3. Certified Coding Specialist (CCS):

Certification Body: American Health Information Management Association (AHIMA)

Website: https://www.ahima.org/certification-careers/certification-exams

Although not specific to revenue cycle management, the CCS certification offered by AHIMA validates expertise in medical coding, which is a critical component of RCM. The certification demonstrates proficiency in assigning accurate codes and ensuring compliance with coding guidelines. AHIMA's website provides details on eligibility, exam content, and study resources for the CCS certification.

4. Certified Professional Coder (CPC):

Certification Body: American Academy of Professional Coders (AAPC)

Website: https://www.aapc.com/certification/cpc/

The CPC certification is offered by AAPC and focuses on medical coding proficiency. Although not RCM-specific, it is relevant for professionals involved in coding processes within the revenue cycle. The certification demonstrates proficiency in CPT, ICD, and HCPCS coding systems. The AAPC website provides information on eligibility requirements, exam details, and study resources for the CPC certification.

These certifications are well-recognized in the healthcare industry and demonstrate proficiency and knowledge in specific areas of revenue cycle management. They can enhance career prospects, validate expertise, and provide a competitive edge in the job market. It is recommended to review the eligibility requirements, exam details, and study resources provided by the respective certification bodies to determine the most suitable certification based on your career goals and experience.

Here are some upcoming conferences, seminars, and events focused on revenue cycle management (RCM):

1. HFMA Annual Conference:

   Date: TBA (typically held in June)

   Website: https://www.hfma.org/conferences/annual-conference/

   The HFMA Annual Conference, organized by the Healthcare Financial Management Association (HFMA), is one of the largest gatherings of healthcare finance and RCM professionals. The conference features keynote speakers, educational sessions, networking opportunities, and an exhibition hall showcasing the latest industry solutions.

2. HBMA Healthcare Revenue Cycle Conference:

   Date: TBA (typically held in September)

   Website: https://www.hbma.org/education/conferences/hrcc

   The Healthcare Revenue Cycle Conference, hosted by the Healthcare Business Management Association (HBMA), focuses on revenue cycle management best practices, regulatory updates, and industry trends. The conference offers educational sessions, roundtable discussions, and networking opportunities.

3. MGMA Annual Conference:

   Date: TBA (typically held in October)

   Website: https://www.mgma.com/events/annual-conference

   The MGMA Annual Conference, organized by the Medical Group Management Association (MGMA), brings together healthcare leaders and professionals to discuss challenges and strategies in medical practice management, including revenue cycle management. The conference offers educational sessions, keynote presentations, and networking events.

4. AHIMA Conference:

   Date: TBA (typically held in September or October)

Website: https://www.ahima.org/events/annual-convention

The AHIMA Conference, organized by the American Health Information Management Association (AHIMA), focuses on health information management, including topics related to coding, documentation, compliance, and revenue cycle management. The conference features educational sessions, expert speakers, and networking opportunities.

5. Becker's Hospital Review RCM + RevTech Virtual Event:

Date: TBA

Website: https://www.beckershospitalreview.com/rcm-revtech-virtual-event/

Becker's Hospital Review hosts virtual events that bring together revenue cycle leaders and technology experts to discuss innovative strategies, technological advancements, and best practices in RCM. The virtual event includes panel discussions, keynote presentations, and networking opportunities.

Please note that event dates and formats may change, so it is recommended to visit the respective websites for the latest information, registration details, speakers, and topics covered. Additionally, there are often regional and local conferences and seminars that focus on RCM, so it is worth exploring industry-specific events in your area for additional learning and networking opportunities.

Here are some online repositories or databases where students can access real-life case studies related to revenue cycle management (RCM):

1. HFMA Case Studies:

   Website: https://www.hfma.org/topics/case-studies/

   The Healthcare Financial Management Association (HFMA) offers a collection of case studies that cover various aspects of revenue cycle management. These case studies provide practical examples, insights into industry challenges, and best practices.

2. MGMA Case Studies:

   Website: https://www.mgma.com/resources/learning-solutions/case-studies

   The Medical Group Management Association (MGMA) provides a series of case studies that focus on revenue cycle management and medical practice management. These case studies offer real-life scenarios, problem-solving approaches, and lessons learned.

3. AHIMA Case Studies:

   Website: https://www.ahima.org/practice-resources/tools-and-resources/case-studies/

   AHIMA offers case studies that cover a wide range of health information management topics, including coding, documentation, compliance, and revenue cycle management. These case studies provide practical examples and insights into industry challenges.

4. Change Healthcare Case Studies:

   Website: https://www.changehealthcare.com/resource-library/case-studies

   Change Healthcare offers a collection of case studies that highlight successful revenue cycle management strategies and outcomes. These case studies showcase real-world scenarios and practical solutions implemented by healthcare organizations.

5. HIMSS Case Studies:

Website: https://www.himss.org/case-studies

The Healthcare Information and Management Systems Society (HIMSS) provides case studies that focus on health information technology and its impact on revenue cycle management. These case studies offer insights into the implementation of technology solutions and their effect on RCM.

Please note that some of these resources may require registration or membership to access the case studies. Additionally, academic institutions, professional associations, and industry publications may also provide case studies relevant to revenue cycle management as part of their educational resources.

With this, we conclude the comprehensive guide to revenue cycle management. I hope this book provides you with valuable knowledge and skills in your journey into this field.

Don't forget to look at the novels and other books on different subjects by the author, VIRUTI SHIVAN, www.mahadev.me. You might find them interesting and life-changing.

Good luck!